Infections and T
A Historical Perspective

Infections and Their Control
A Historical Perspective

Dr SWB Newsom

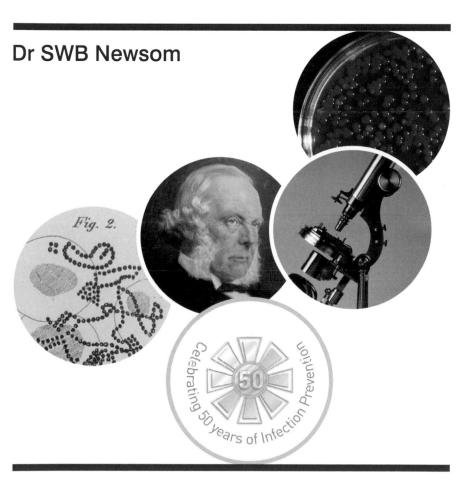

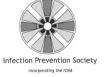

Infection Prevention Society
Incorporating the ICNA

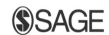

Los Angeles | London | New Delhi
Singapore | Washington DC

First published 2009

SAGE Publications Ltd
1 Oliver's Yard
55 City Road
London EC1Y 1SP

SAGE Publications Inc.
2455 Teller Road
Thousand Oaks, California 91320

SAGE Publications India Pvt Ltd
B 1/I 1 Mohan Cooperative Industrial Area
Mathura Road, Post Bag 7
New Delhi 110 044

SAGE Publications Asia-Pacific Pte Ltd
33 Pekin Street #02-01
Far East Square
Singapore 048763

British Library Cataloguing in Publication data

A catalogue record for this book is available from the British Library

ISBN 978-1-84920-453-8

Typeset by C&M Digitals (P) Ltd, Chennai, India
Printed in Great Britain by Ashford Colour Press Ltd
Printed on paper from sustainable resources

To celebrate the 50th Anniversary of the first Infection Control Nurse in England.

In 1959 on-site assistance and advice were needed by surgeons in Torbay, and with matron's permission, they appointed an ICN (Infection Control Nurse). The outcome was successful enough to justify publication in *The Lancet*, and the name of Brendan Moore, the Exeter microbiologist, has passed into infection control 'lore' as a parent of the ICN.

In 1963, Stanford University appointed Kathryn Wenzel as the first ICN in the USA.

Contents

Foreword

In ancient times, infection was often considered to be due to malevolence of evil spirits, witchcraft or the wrath of god or later to the corruption of the air caused by climate changes. More 'scientific' theories gradually emerged, the most important being the presence of miasmas consisting of putrid air arising from decaying animal and vegetable matter or stagnant water and cesspools. Contagion (spread by emanation from an infected patient) was later recognised in leprosy and plague before the isolation and identification of living organisms in the late 19th century.

Dr SWB (Bill) Newsom's series of articles begins mainly at this stage, although hygiene in the days of the ancient Romans is also included. The series provides a wealth of information on the life and work of eminent workers in the field of infection. Of particular interest is that that so many of their colleagues did not initially accept their conclusions even when good evidence was provided. This difficulty with control of infection has continued to some extent up to the present time.

Bill Newsom has always had a particular interest in methods of sterilisation and he gives an interesting account of their development over the years. He was personally involved in the practical aspects of ensuring that the use of sterilisers in hospital was reliable and safe, and was an active member of BSI and Department of Health committees on sterilisation and decontamination, a longtime member and past secretary of the Central Sterilising Club and a past President of the Institute of Decontamination Sciences as well as a past President of the Hospital Infection Society.

The evidence that infections were caused by living organisms and disproving the theory of spontaneous generation by Louis Pasteur in the late 19th century was one of the main advances in medicine. At about the same time Robert Koch and his colleagues identified the causative organisms of most bacterial diseases by laboratory methods which are still in use today. Koch was probably the greatest bacteriologist of all time and many bacteria were named after his co-workers or assistants. Both Koch and Pasteur realised the importance of killing bacteria and introduced decontamination by heat, e.g. pasteurisation, and the use of steam in Koch's 'steriliser', which was used in laboratories until recently. Koch also recognised the problem of killing spores. However, before Pasteur and Koch identified living organisms as causes of infection, the importance of handwashing was recognised by several doctors and it's value in preventing transmission of infection in maternity patients in Vienna was shown by Semmelweiss in one of the first clinical trials of hand disinfection. However, doctors at the time refused to accept that death of patients could be due to their deficient practices and the results of his studies were not accepted by his head of department as well as many of his colleagues.

Florence Nightingale was known to the general public as 'the lady with the lamp' in the Crimean War, but despite many years of suffering from 'Crimean fever' (possibly brucellosis), followed by a chronic depressive disease, her achievements were immense as a nurse administrator, a statistician, a hospital architect, a nurse educator and public health expert. She was a great believer in cleanliness and good ventilation, but not contagion, and never accepted the germ theory of disease. She was well known nationally and was included in a chapter of Lytton Strachey's book on 'Eminent Victorians'. Another major figure was Joseph Lister who was the first surgeon to be given a peerage. He studied the work of Pasteur on fermentation and putrefaction and subsequently developed the use of disinfectants to prevent wound infection in surgery. Although a number of surgeons did not agree with his methods, his reduction in post-operative mortality was impressive and led to the aseptic techniques of the 20th century. About the same time, Alexander Ogston, an Aberdeen surgeon, described staphylococci and streptococci in pus from infected wounds.

Sewage in the streets and rivers had long been recognised as a probable source of enteral infections, but John Snow showed that contaminated drinking water was the main hazard. His removal of the handle of the pump which supplied well water in Broad Street was followed by a reduction in cholera by users of the pump. Vaccination against smallpox by Lady Mary Wortley Montague and later by Edward Jenner, as well as the identification of tuberculosis, typhoid fever, and poliomyelitis by other eminent physicians are also described and there is an interesting article on the development of the microscope, which included the work of Lister's father, who presented his famous son with an up- to-date microscope.

Bill Newsom's interest in brucellosis developed when he acquired the infection as a child and was treated with M & B 693, an early sulphonamide. Surprisingly his infection responded to this treatment. The restored laboratory of David Bruce and the Maltese bacteriologist, Dr Zammit, the discoverers of *Brucella melitensis*, can still be seen in Valetta and is well worth a visit.

The discovery of penicillin by Alexander Fleming in 1929 and its development as a clinical agent by Florey, Chain and colleagues was followed by the discovery of a number of other antibiotics during the 1940s to the 1960s. It was suggested by some bacteriologists that penicillin provided the elimination of bacterial infections, as a major clinical problem specially staphylococci. As a consequence, the aseptic methods developed at the beginning of the 20th century were thought by many surgeons to have become redundant, but bacteria such as

Staphylococcus aureus, which have always lived in close contact with man, were able to select appropriate survival mechanisms, and some strains of staphylococci and Gram-negative bacilli are now resistant to most antibiotics. Epidemic strains of MRSA have spread to most countries of the world and control is often difficult and expensive. The author's interest in staphylococci started as an adolescent when he developed recurrent boils at a time when penicillin-resistant strains were already spreading in hospitals.

Bill Newsom is an experienced medical microbiologist and research worker, with a long standing interest in the history of bacteriology and infection. He has always stressed the importance of knowledge of the past in dealing with the problems of today. The articles in this book are clear and concise and the diagrams and illustrations and his inclusion of descriptions of his personal experiences are of particular interest. The articles have been published the *British Journal of Intection Control*, to much acclaim. A collection of them all in one book will be a welcome addition to the bookshelf of microbiologists, infection control nurses and others interested in infection.

Graham Ayliffe
Emeritus Professor of Medical Microbiology, University of Birmingham
formerly Director of the Hospital Infection Research Laboratory,
City Hospital, Birmingham

Introduction

'Welcome to my History of Infection Control series' – I wrote these words at the start of my first article, which appeared in June 2001 (Fig 1). Little did I know that eight years later I would have written 27 articles, with more in prospect. I aimed to write about the people and events that contributed to the foundation of our work. I found some fascinating stories, and have travelled to Budapest, Vienna, Rome, Malta, and around the UK in search of material.

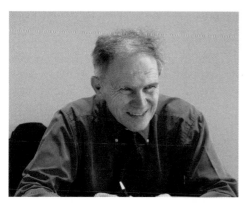

Figure 1   The Author (M. Greig)

I can still remember the evening when as a student I opened my first textbook of bacteriology (now a valuable antique) and became so immersed that it was 2 a.m. before I stopped reading, having completed half the text. It must have been an omen – for it was the introduction to a very happy professional life. Do not worry – I am not going to keep you up all night, but I hope you will enjoy reading about some of our predecessors and their problems.

I am very grateful to the successive editors of the Journal, and also to Matthew Pulzer its previous publisher, for encouragement, and for suggesting challenging titles – 'Microscopes' and 'Romans' spring to mind. A big THANK YOU to SAGE Publications and Tracy Cooper when editor for the idea of putting them together; and to Graham Ayliffe, Past President of the ICNA, for his Foreword. Like the rest of the world I always knew I could turn to him for advice when infection control problems got too much, and was very pleased to follow him in various national roles. One of my treasures is a reprint request from the US Army for a joint paper addressed to 'The Hospital Infection Research Centre, Birmingham, Papworth Hospital, Cambridge'. I spent many hours under his chairmanship of the Department of Health's Microbiology Advisory Committee, and was also grateful to the Department of Health for 18 years support for my researches into engineering aspects of hospital design and equipment.

Life is cyclic. Now, long since retired, I live only three miles from my student room, with the university library nearby (much used both today and as a student). This project revived my interest in history and kept my brain moving. It prompted me to review my childhood illnesses (before the advent of antibiotics – when treatment of a sore throat was painting with tincture of iodine – very painful), together with my working lives in London, Hong Kong, and Papworth/ Addenbrooke's.

The Papworth Laboratory was originally named The Sims Woodhead Memorial Laboratory in honour of its founder the Cambridge Professor of Pathology. Sims Woodhead was the author of the first British textbook of bacteriology, *Bacteria and their Products* (1891) (Fig 2).

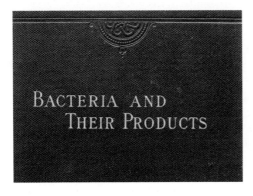

In it he described: tuberculosis, cholera, typhoid fever, leprosy, actinomycosis, anthrax, tetanus, diphtheria, and hydrophobia (rabies), many of which appear in my articles. His chapter on tuberculosis is very detailed and his finding of tubercle bacilli in milk, antedates the Royal Commission on bovine tuberculosis (of which he became a member) by 20 years.

He provided an interesting paragraph on infection control:

Figure 2   Sims Woodhead's Book

'By far the best disinfectant is moist heat' … various chemicals are mentioned – but 'none of these can, for a moment, be compared as regards not only efficiency and cheapness, but also for ease of use, with steam or boiling water'. 'No room that has been occupied by a pthisical (tuberculous) patient should be used until it has been disinfected; the bedding and curtains should be well boiled, the blankets steamed, all the furniture washed with soap and water, the carpets and upholstery thoroughly beaten in the open air over straw, which should then be burned, the floor thoroughly washed with soap and water, and the wallpaper rubbed down with freshly baked bread (used even to-day to clean leaves in books!)' … as a final comment he writes 'In San Remo all these methods have been brought to the notice of hotel keepers, and they are advised to use them for all rooms at the end of each season, not only the sleeping rooms, but also the public rooms'.

For 1891 – only a few years after the discovery of tubercle bacilli – this shows a remarkably modern approach.

My own attempts at providing infection control services in the 1970s–1980s were frustrating. Throughout East Anglia, isolation rooms in new hospitals were not commissioned on the grounds that 'infectious disease' – measles and the like – was a thing of the past. Half of the Cambridge infectious disease ward was turned over to haematology. When a new hospital for Huntingdon was planned – the Matron (yes!) in Cambridge agreed to a second infection control nurse, as our existing one had to cover Cambridge (three hospitals), Papworth, Huntingdon, Ely and Newmarket. However by the time Huntingdon hospital was commissioned, it came under a different administration. What do you want an infection control nurse for? asked the surgeons – wishing to extend their empire. In the end we got a half time nurse, who spent the rest of her time in Occupational Health. Later we had a dedicated part-time nurse, whose sessions I supplemented from my research funds, and finally made whole-time with money provided for AIDS. Today new hospitals are being planned with many isolation rooms, and the Papworth/ Huntingdon set-up has four infection control nurses with a fifth in prospect. I don't know whether to be glad that I was on the right track, or sorry that it has taken the onslaught of MRSA and *Clostridium difficile* to bring this about.

The articles did not appear in a planned way, although some followed on naturally. I have taken the opportunity to rationalise their order. As handwashing remains the number one priority – we start with Semmelweis (for a dramatic account of his life try: *The Cry and the Covenant* by Morton Thompson – 'brilliantly described semi-fiction'). My articles on Florence Nightingale follow on; like Semmelweis, her main work was done when bacteria had not been defined as the cause of 'contagion'. A visit to the Florence Nightingale museum at St. Thomas' Hospital is well worthwhile – and since writing my articles I have heard a lecture on Russian medical services in the Crimea (by a Professor of Medical History from Moscow). The famous Surgeon Nikolai Ivanovich Pirogof is credited with the first full use of 'triage' and the provision of an excellent medical service – he was backed up by the 'Sisters of Charity', a team of nurses. Indeed the knowledge of their existence may have contributed to the invitation to Florence to go to Scutari.

Lister also commenced work before bacteria had been defined, but became interested in Pasteur's findings, and became the first person to grow bacteria in pure culture. He was more interested in the concept of bacteria than their type and it was left to Ogston to relate staphylococci to wound infection and abscesses. However Robert Koch really put medical microbiology on the map, inventing techniques, growing bacteria and relating them to disease. 1882 is the 1066 of medical microbiology – the year he grew the tubercle bacillus. Although Pasteur's works largely antedate Koch's, his work ties things together. Although this was the 1800s, it was amazing how much interaction went on between the three, with Lister inviting Koch to London to demonstrate his techniques, and Pasteur watching on

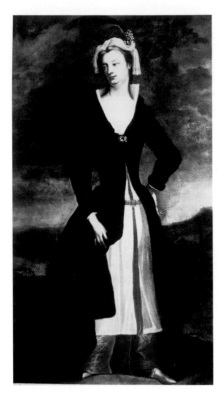

Figure 3 Lady Mary Wortley Montagu (National Gallery of Ireland)

approvingly. Later however Pasteur and Koch had great disagreements.

The description of microscopes allows me to show Lister's father's work, and is followed by two papers on vaccination – the first describing my heroine (again from my student days) – Lady Mary Wortley Montagu, whose portrait hangs in the National Gallery of Ireland in Dublin (Fig 3). Sims Woodhead quotes Lady Mary's letter of 23 March 1718 from Belgrade: 'the boy (her son) was ingrafted last Tuesday, and is at this time singing and playing, impatient for his supper. I pray to God my next letter may give as good an account of him' (it did). The second paper presents the better known story of Edward Jenner who perhaps did more than anyone to prevent infectious diseases. Both episodes show the ability of people to make observations, and then to capitalise on them. A visit to the Jenner Museum in Berkeley provides a worthwhile day out, with the possibility of visits to Slimbridge, or to Berkeley Castle for those interested in birds or history.

The Romans were well advanced in provision of water supplies and sewage disposal as well as roads. However the thought of 1500 bathing at a time in the baths of Caracalla certainly creates concern. The article on Rome serves to introduce infections that are waterborne, or with faecal-oral spread: cholera, legionnaires disease, typhoid and polio. There are some marvellous detective stories. John Snow stands out as his work, like that of Semmelweis and Florence Nightingale, preceded the concept of bacteria. Interestingly enough Sims Woodhead, who wrote a long chapter on cholera, does not mention Snow at all. Several other early English textbooks of bacteriology also ignored Snow's work – presumably because it didn't describe the bacteria. Once Koch had grown the bacteria–his work on epidemiology was quoted *in extenso* in preference to that of Snow.

Polio was always a favourite topic of mine, stimulated by the thought that I had probably had a non-paralytic infection at school. I have a long standing interest in the vaccine following a student project on it, at a time when it was all happening (in the 1950s). The polio story reflects three aspects of human behaviour. Firstly it was a disease of civilisation. Before proper sewage disposal it was so universal that newborn babies were infected, but did not develop disease because of protection from mother's antibodies. As the world became more hygienic, so babies were no longer infected, but older children, who had no innate immunity, became affected – and the disease increased to epidemic proportions. Secondly the power of a community working together to overcome a problem was well illustrated by the 'March of Dimes' in the USA. Thirdly, sadly international distrust has delayed the perfectly possible goal of eradicating polio (a purely human disease) from the world by vaccination.

My visit to Malta was greatly enhanced by Michael Borg, Chairman of IFIC, who took me to see the restored laboratory where Zammit first related brucellosis to goats. Zammit appears in my article only as 'The Government Bacteriologist', but visitors to Malta will see his work everywhere – not least in the Valetta Museum for he became a famous archaeologist and head of the university, summed up in the dedication of a book on Malta written in 1912 by Bradley (Fig 4).

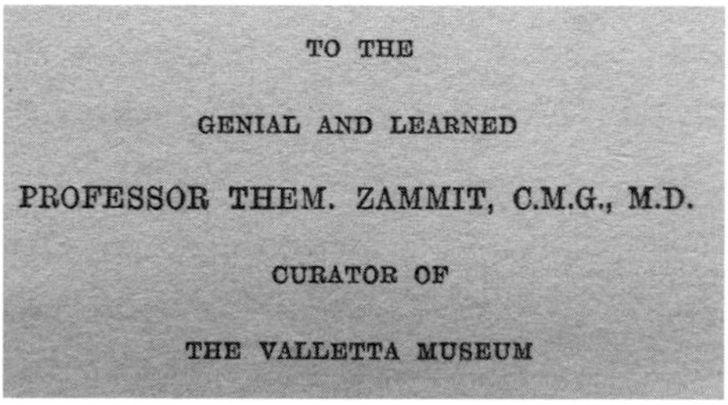

Brucellosis (from fresh cows milk – courtesy of my grandmother) made me quite ill. However like 50% of children

TO THE

GENIAL AND LEARNED

PROFESSOR THEM. ZAMMIT, C.M.G., M.D.

CURATOR OF

THE VALLETTA MUSEUM

Figure 4   A dedication (Newsom)

from the 1930s I had tuberculosis without knowing it – purely a positive mantoux test as a medical student. Most of my working life I thought TB was on the way out – but alas no more. While writing this article, I have taken time out to view articles submitted to the *Journal of Hospital Infection* from Brazil, and from South Korea, on infection control for phthisic (can you remember this word?) patients.

As always – life with the staphylococci moves on. While I mentioned their production of Leucocidin, I didn't burden you with the second Leucocidin – discovered by Panton and Valentine. Now shortened to PVL – strains producing it have become worrying enough to warrant: 'Guidance on the diagnosis and management of PVL-associated *Staphylococcus aureus* infections (PVL-SA) in the UK' – issued by the Health Protection Agency (edited by me!). Another recent publication of note is: 'Superbugs and Superdrugs: A History of MRSA.' This is a transcript of an afternoon spent in recollections of MRSA, by people associated with its progress as part of the 'Wellcome Witnesses to Twentieth Century Medicine' series (you may recognise one of my illustrations in it!).

I have given a few key references under the heading of 'Further Reading'. Most are books, and I can thoroughly recommend searching on www.abebooks.com (cheapest first) or even e-bay, as many of them can be bought for a modest few pounds.

All in all I have had a lot of fun doing these articles, and have been very pleased by the response I have had – to my albeit relaxed approach. I have tried to make them personalised, and been fortunate that my working life has encompassed so many of the topics I have written about – although less so when it came to suffering the infections myself. I look forward to writing some more. I am always open to suggestion for new topics although whether there will be enough for a second volume remains to be seen.

Many people have helped by providing me with illustrations – in particular I wish to thank The Wellcome Foundation (Wellcome Images), The Nuffield Foundation, The Royal College of Surgeons (London), Professor Thomas Brock, and The Jenner Museum for multiple pictures.

I am grateful to the National Gallery of Ireland for permission to reproduce Figure 3.

Chapter 1
Semmelweis and Handwashing

Introduction

The single most important factor in prevention of infection in hospitals is hand hygiene, and the person who gets the credit for ramming this home was Hungarian – Ignaz Philip Semmelweis.

Semmelweis was born in Buda in 1818. The son of a prosperous merchant: his house still stands between the castle and the river, and is now a Museum of the History of Medicine (which is well worth a visit). He wanted to study medicine and at the time Vienna Medical School was the world 'centre of excellence' and so off he went to the capital of the Austro-Hungarian empire and by 1844 aged 26 he had obtained the MD.

As a student he was lucky enough to have some excellent teachers of scientific method – Rokitansky the morbid anatomist (credited with over 30,000 autopsies) and Skoda (the inventor of auscultation). The messages were: gather the data, formulate a hypothesis, and then test it. When he qualified he opted for obstetrics and went to work as an unpaid 'Aspirant' (houseman) to the post of 'Assistant' (Registrar) to Professor Klein – the very autocratic and powerful professor of obstetrics – appointed by the Emperor himself to look after the royal family.

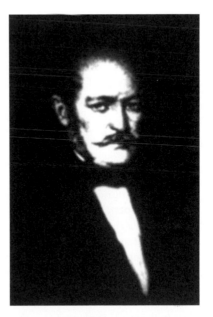

Figure 1   Ignaz Philip Semmelweis (1818–1865) (Allgemeine Krankenhaus, Vienna)

The problem

At the time there were three obstetric wards in the university hospital (the Allgemeine Krankenhaus): The First Division, which was run by medical students: the Second Division run by midwives and a secret one for the professor's use! Klein had abandoned the methods of his predecessor (who had studied in Dublin and had notions of hygiene) and made the students practise on the patients rather than with a leather model 'baby'.

When Semmelweis started work he was appalled to find that mothers attending the First Division had a horrific death rate (22.5% in November 1841). They died of 'childbed' fever (now known to be streptococcal blood poisoning).

The students attended autopsies all morning and practised on the bodies, so much so that when they went on the ward afterwards to examine the patients their clothes smelt of the dead.

The search for clues to the cause occupied Semmelweis for several years (remember that bacteria were not yet known about). Klein had an 'atmospheric, cosmic, telluric' theory, whatever that meant: but if so why did it affect only one of the divisions? The Second with its lower mortality acted as a 'control'.

Overcrowding could not have been the cause because the mothers desperately tried to be placed in the Second Division, and anyway the First was larger. The same linen was used and the same corridors. The only real difference was that the medical students delivered babies in the First Division and the midwives in the Second.

A ban on overseas students did no good, nor did a reduction in student numbers. Altering the way in which the priest went round preceded by the Sacristan ringing his bell to administer the last rites was equally useless. Semmelweis did manage to silence the bell. He wrote: 'One can imagine what an impression the sound of the little bell made on the mothers, as for myself it made me uneasy of spirit … a sigh stole from my breast for the new victim who had fallen beneath this unknown cause'. The little bell was an agonising reminder to reinvestigate the cause with all zeal possible.

Clues

Semmelweis found several clues. The long labour in mothers having their first baby – identified as 'blooming young girls teeming with health' – was all too often a risk factor: then there were the 'street-births' who were admitted free, often so the newborn baby could be adopted. These numbered up to 100 per month, but remained well despite the primitive surroundings of the birth, and those admitted with a premature labour were also 'low risk'.

One other clue was that patients were often struck down in relation to their place in the ward – beds next to each other were risk factors – something that did not happen in the Second Division. Two years later (in the winter of 1846) Semmelweis had collected vast amounts of data, including masses of monthly mortality statistics comparing the two Divisions, but failed to come up with a sensible hypothesis.

Klein meanwhile had not been very pleased to see his houseman's interference, and although he promoted Semmelweis when the Registrar came to the end of his two-year contract, promotion only lasted a few months and then his predecessor was re-employed (an unheard-of event) and Semmelweis was sacked.

The discovery

Undaunted, Semmelweis did some laboratory work on rabbits with vaginal secretions from dead mothers, and learnt English in preparation for a visit to Dublin. However, his predecessor suddenly got a professor's job and so Semmelweis was recalled to the Allgemeine Krankenhaus

Before taking up his post again, he went to Venice for a short holiday. While he was away the assistant pathologist Dr Kolletschka (a close friend) had his arm jostled by one of the students while doing an autopsy on a newly dead mother. He cut himself and three days later was dead.

Later Semmelweis wrote of his return from Vienna 'still animated by my visit to the Venetian treasure houses, still more agitated by the report of Kolletschka's death, there was forced on my mind with irresistible clarity the identity of this disease with that of so many mothers. In Kolletschka the specific cause was cadaver particles, which were introduced into his vascular system ... the staff and students have frequent contact with cadavers. That the cadaveric particles are not entirely removed by normal washing with soap is shown by the continuing cadaveric odour. During examination of patients, the hand contaminated with cadaveric particles is brought into contact with the genitals allowing absorption into the vascular system'. What an horrific discovery – he himself had doubtless caused many deaths.

The proof

Semmelweis conducted 'three trials' to test the hypothesis. In May 1847 he made all staff and students wash their hands in 'chlorina liquida' (known to be a disinfectant), and later changed this to chlorinated lime as it was cheaper. The mortality dropped from 11.4% to 3% (see Figure 2).

However, corpses were not the sole source of 'cadaveric particles'. A woman in labour with a 'foully discharging leg cancer' was put in the first bed of the ward. Staff only washed with soap and water after examining her, and subsequently eleven of the 12 women delivered along with her died. Thus an 'ichorous discharge' from living organisms (in this case human) was also dangerous, and this lesson was hammered home when a woman with a 'carious' (infected) knee joint also acted as a source of fatal infections for others on the ward, possibly by airborne spread of infection.

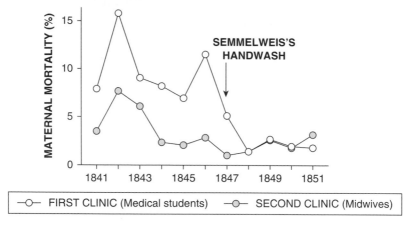

Figure 2   Maternal mortality at the Allgemeine Krankenhaus, showing the drop following Semmelweis's introduction of handwashing (M. Rotter)

Interlude

1847 was a turbulent year with revolution afoot in the Empire – indeed Semmelweis put on his uniform and marched with the Academic Legion – which was no great problem as the university had been closed down. When he returned to work, he resumed experiments with the rabbits.

Semmelweis regarded his discovery as a revelation that was so self-evident it did not need publicity. He was deeply disturbed to find this was not the case – many did not believe him. One prominent doctor said: 'We should wait [for a definite knowledge of the disease] and wash.'

Semmelweis did not like writing and so it was 13 years before he finally wrote his book on 'Kindbettfiebers'. However, the professor, who was livid at being criticised, had won out. Semmelweis's job ended and he could not get a career job in Vienna, while his pathological collaborator was thrown into jail for helping the rebels. He left in high dudgeon for home in 1849 saying he would never return to Vienna and eventually became Professor of Obstetrics in Pest.

Final proof and later years

In Pest he applied his principles satisfactorily, but did have one outbreak of childbed that was traced to an economical matron not changing sheets between patients, so that the 'cadaveric particles' were again being spread around. The outbreak was terminated by laundering.

Thus Semmelweis had now defined the disease, and found at least three modes of spread: hands, air, and dirty linen. He concluded that childbed fever depended on absorption of decomposed animal matter, which caused a disintegration of the blood.

The opposition to his theory hurt him terribly. By the time he finally published his book in 1861 (see Figure 3), he was an embittered man and although the book has the statistics and proof, it rambles on and in it he accuses some eminent professors of being murderers. Indeed controversy still surrounds his discovery, but the international community paid due respect to him later by erecting a statue outside the hospital in Pest, where it still stands (see Figure 4).

Some years later Billroth (better known as inventor of an operation to remove the stomach), also in Vienna, actually saw and described strepto cocci (from a wound exudate). Visitors to Vienna should make for the small Museum of the History of Medicine, in which Semmelweis's washbasin (see Figure 5) and Billroth's microscope can be seen.

By 1865 Semmelweis was showing definite signs of mental illness. His wife finally suggested a 'holiday' in Vienna where he was met by a friend and transported to a mental hospital. Within six weeks he was dead of streptococcal blood poisoning, said to have been acquired from a wound in his hand while doing an operation.

Whatever the truth, the final irony was that the body was returned to the Allgemeine Krankenhaus for autopsy.

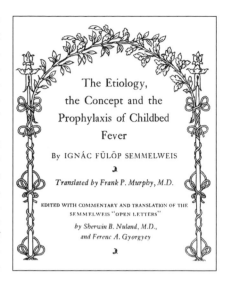

The Etiology,
the Concept and the
Prophylaxis of Childbed
Fever

By IGNÁC FÜLÖP SEMMELWEIS

Translated by Frank P. Murphy, M.D.

EDITED WITH COMMENTARY AND TRANSLATION OF THE
SEMMELWEIS "OPEN LETTERS"

by Sherwin B. Nuland, M.D.,
and Ferenc A. Gyorgyey

Figure 3 Semmelweis finally published his book in 1831 after years of criticism by the medical establishment; recent translation (Newsom)

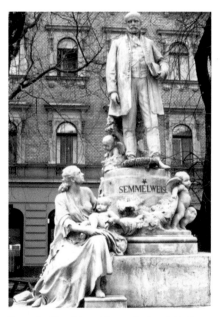

Figure 4 The statue of Semmelweis outside the hospital in Budapest (Newsom)

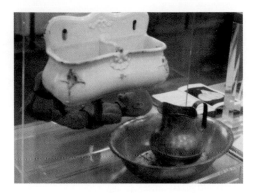

Figure 5   Semmelweis's washbasin survives intact and may be seen at the Museum of the History of Medicine (Newsom)

Acknowledgements

I am grateful to Prof. Manfred Rotter for Figure 1 and the Allgemeine Frankenhaus for Figure 2.

Further reading

Dormandy Thomas. 'Semmelweis and Childbed Fever' in *Moments of Truth*. Chichester, John Wiley, 2003.

de Kruif Paul. 'Semmelweis saver of mothers' in *Men Against Death*. London, Jonathan Cape, 1933.

Newsom SWB. Ignaz Philip Semmelweis. *Journal of Hospital Infection*. **23**, 175–187.

Thompson Morton. *The Cry and the Covenant*. New York, Doubleday, 1949 (an over-dramatised version).

Chapter 2
Florence Nightingale part 1: 1820–1856

Introduction

Although Florence Nightingale referred to prevention of 'zymotic' diseases, she did all her relevant work before the germ theory of infection – a theory she never really took seriously. Nevertheless, she was the first to state many of the principles we use today.

Florence Nightingale was born in 1820, two years after Semmelweis and seven years before Lister. In her lifetime she became a national heroine, reforming the sanitary conditions of the army (especially in India), designing hospitals, and founding a famous nurse training school.

Like many Victorians she kept copies of most of her 13,000 letters, and so her life is exceptionally well documented. The scope of her achievements and the data available means that there is easily enough material for two articles – even when restricting discussion just to infection control.

INTRODUCTORY NOTES
ON
LYING-IN INSTITUTIONS.

TOGETHER WITH

A PROPOSAL FOR
ORGANISING AN INSTITUTION FOR TRAINING MIDWIVES
AND MIDWIFERY NURSES.

BY

FLORENCE NIGHTINGALE.

LONDON:
LONGMANS, GREEN, AND CO.
1871.

Figure 1   Florence Nightingale's booklets were most influential (Newsom)

Three of her booklets are particularly relevant to the history of infection control: *Notes on Hospitals* (1859, 1863). *Notes on Nursing* (1860), and *Introductory Notes on Lying-in Institutions* (1871) (see Figure 1). Cecil

Woodham Smith wrote a comprehensive biography in 1970, and a biography with selected letters is presented in *Ever yours. Florence Nightingale*, edited by Martha Vicinus and Bea Nergaard.

Other biographies abound, including a well-illustrated one by Elspeth Huxley (all can be purchased secondhand for £10 to £15 through the websites: www.abebooks.co.uk or www.amazon.co.uk)

Early life

Nightingale's parents were rich enough to have an extended honeymoon in Italy and since Florence was the name of the town in which she was born her parents settled on this for her (her elder sister had been born two years earlier in Naples and so was called Parthenope, from Parthe).

On their return to England the family eventually settled in two houses: Embley (now a boys school) on the edge of the New Forest (for winter) and Lea Hurst (now a Royal Surgical Aid Society home) in Derbyshire. 'It had only 15 bedrooms', said Florence, 'so it cannot be called a large house'.

The Nightingales' daughters were expected to stay at home, look after their parents and prepare to become good 'Victorian wives'.

Florence, however, volunteered to nurse other members of their large family when ill or having babies, and visited the sick and needy in the village. She travelled extensively on the continent, and whenever the opportunity arose she visited hospitals. As befitted the daughter of an upper-class family she was presented at court. Her father, who had a good (but in her view underused) brain, arranged for the girls to have lessons at home – teaching Latin, German, French, Italian, history and philosophy himself. Nightingale preferred mathematics, which she thought would be more useful and studied almost in secret. 'What use are mathematics to a married woman?' said her mother. She was not short of suitors – her cousin Henry proposed to her, and more to the point Richard Monkton Miles, poet and philosopher, courted her for seven years. However, aged 17 Nightingale had had a revelation – God had called her to do something as yet undetermined, but special, and she was saving herself for this.

Throughout her 20s she was an increasingly rebellious young woman, kept firmly in tow by her family. She made influential friends and became more and more drawn to nursing.

The state of British health care in the 1840s was appalling. The more affluent were nursed at home, although usually by relatives without medical training, while the nurses in the few public hospitals were usually of low quality, and even alcoholic; satirised as Sairey Gamp in Charles Dickens' *Martin Chuzzlewit*. Religious orders tended to provide better quality nurses, although as Nightingale found out later there could be friction between different religions.

A visit to Rome

Early in 1848 (when Semmelweis was involved in revolution) Nightingale visited Rome, where she met Sir Sidney Herbert and Elizabeth his wife, who were to become prime figures in her life.

She hoped to persuade her family to let her visit Kaiserworth, a religious institution on the Rhine, where she could train for nursing in secure surroundings. The family, however, objected. Nightingale bottled up her frustration, which was slightly assuaged by a secret visit there for a fortnight in 1849.

However, she did achieve permission for three months' training later in the following year – while Parthe was in Carlsbad for a 'cure'. The cost was looking after Parthe at home for the next six months, which she found extremely difficult. Family frustrations continued, but in 1853 Nightingale (aged 33) finally cast herself adrift in a reasonably acceptable way by becoming Superintendent of the Harley Street Hospital for Gentlewomen on the recommendation of Elizabeth Herbert.

Her father gave her an allowance of £500 a year and in preparation she went to learn about nursing in Paris from the Sisters of Charity – a visit cut short by measles.

Learning to influence

The job was a good introduction to her real strength – administration. Her letter to the chair of the governors from Paris is full of sensible details. 'The carrying of hot water all over the house is desirable. The cheapest way of doing it is, I believe, to have a boiler at the top of the house with a small fire to heat it...'

She became an expert in manipulating committees. To her father she wrote: 'Now I perceive I do all my business by intrigue. I propose to A, B or C the resolution I think they are most capable of carrying in committee and leave it to them, and I always win.' Although she did a lot of nursing, administration loomed large – the accounts were in disarray, and she soon developed a proper accounting system.

Around this time the writer Mrs Gaskell described her as: 'tall; very slight and willowy in figure... grey eyes, which are generally pensive and drooping, but which when they choose can be the merriest eyes I ever saw... She has a great deal of fun, and is carried along by that I think. She mimics most capitally'.

One delightful (although not strictly relevant) story is of Athena the owl, rescued by Nightingale as a baby from children in Athens and brought home in need

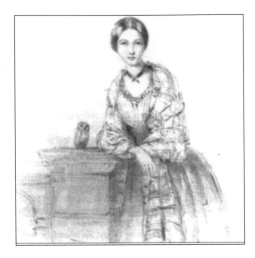

Figure 2   Florence Nightingale with Athena the owl (Bridgeman Art Library)

of nursing. A letter to her mother noted: 'Athena is better, by dint of a daily bird.' Sadly in the hurly burly of packing for the Crimea. Athena got locked in an attic and did not recover, but her memory endured (see Figure 2).

The shock of Crimea

By the summer of 1854 Nightingale had become more experienced and her mentors were suggesting more challenging jobs, such as Nurse Superintendent at Kings College Hospital, with scope for nurse training.

However, fate intervened in October with reports from William Russell in *The Times* on the war against Russia. The reports, made much more immediate by the telegraph, horrified the nation, notwithstanding efforts from the War Office to have them toned down. 'It is with surprise and anger,' he wrote, 'that the public will learn that no sufficient preparations have been made for the care of the wounded,' then followed with the details 'men left to perish in agony, unheeded'.

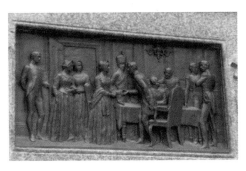

Figure 3   Florence Nightingale offered to take a team of nurses to the Crimea (Newsom)

Two of many reactions were the setting up of a 'Times Fund', and Nightingale's letter to Elizabeth Herbert offering to take a team of nurses to the Crimea. This crossed with a letter from Sir Sidney, now Minister-at-War, asking Nightingale, on behalf of the cabinet, to become the 'Lady Superintendent of Nurses in Turkey' (a later cause of controversy as much of the work was in Russia) (see Figure 3).

She collected 38 nurses and essential supplies and set off four days later, arriving on 4 November at the Barracks Hospital, Scutari (on the Asiatic side of the Bosphorus opposite Istanbul).

Overcoming prejudice

Her position was complex and difficult. She was inserted into the hospital by government decree, but had an independent source of funds (over £30,000).

However, she had no opportunity for consultation with those in authority, either in the War Office or the Crimea. The latter still insisted the situation was acceptable (a situation many infection control practitioners will understand).

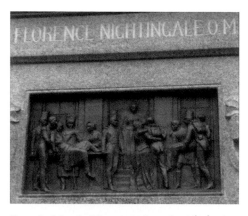

Figure 4   Injured soldiers were often safer at the front than risking a fraught and exhausting journey to the base hospital (Newsom)

The British ambassador to Turkey in Istanbul said there was no need for help and that the Times Fund would be better spent on a church for the English in the city. In fact, conditions were horrendous. In the first seven months of the campaign mortality in the Army was 60% from disease alone.

Paradoxically, ill or wounded soldiers survived better at the front than in the base hospitals. To reach 'professional help' they had to be carried eight miles over mud, spend five days on a ship, and then be carried up to the hospital (see Figure 4).

Frustration and success

When Nightingale's party arrived they were virtually ignored by the hospital doctors, given five small bare rooms as accommodation, and 'locked out' of the wards. However, four days later a flood of patients arrived and prejudices were abandoned.

Nurses began by making beds from sacks stuffed with straw, laid in the wards and corridors, and they dressed wounds. The army supplies, already inefficient, broke down. Patients lacked the basics of life – food, clothing and medicines. Washing for most was allowed once in 80 days. For 1,000 men inactivated with diarrhoea there were 20 chamber pots.

The consequences of all this,' wrote Nightingale to Herbert on 25 November, 'are fever, cholera, gangrene, lice. bugs, fleas and maybe erysipelas – from using one sponge on so many wounds'.

By 10 December a kitchen had been organised, and a 'great deal more cleaning of wards – mops, scrubbing brushes (200 were purchased), brooms and combs – given out by ourselves where not forced from supplies'. The lavatories were unblocked.

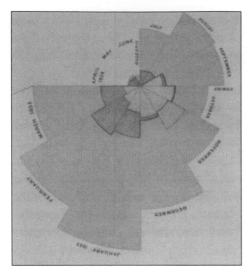

Figure 5   Florence Nightingale was a meticulous collector of data, which she presented in pictorial charts (Bridgeman Art Library)

Drinking water was boiled. The men's clothes were washed. Statistics were collected and later presented as pictorial charts (see Figure 5).

However, the mortality remained unchanged with 1,473 patients dying in the hospital in January 1855, and 1,151 in February. These deaths were largely from illness caught in the hospital, especially cholera, typhus (fleas/rats) and hospital gangrene.

A 'sanitary commission' summoned by Nightingale from Britain in March described the situation as 'murderous'. Beneath the Barrack Hospital lay choked, inefficient sewers, so that the whole building stood in a sea of decaying filth.

Nurses had noted that some beds carried a high mortality, and these were near the doors of privies, where poisonous gases were released from the sewers. The sewers were flushed and cleaned (two dead horses were removed and buried), the ward walls were limewashed, and the shelving which harboured rats, was removed throughout. The effect was instant, deaths from March to May were 418, 169, and 76 respectively.

Nightingale's life became one of complex administration – trying to improve the lot of the soldiers, maintaining discipline among her nurses, and communicating with the army doctors locally, the War Office in London, and her friends and family at home.

She still made time to comfort dying soldiers, write to their relatives, and become 'The Lady with the Lamp'. Despite continuous official disapproval from many quarters she gradually built up a fantastic reputation among the soldiers, their families and the nation in general.

Illness and acclaim

In May, when Scutari had stabilised, Nightingale set off to the Crimea, where there were two hospitals. She was accompanied by Alexis Soyer, one of London's leading chefs, who had come at his own expense to try and improve the patients' diet.

There was fierce opposition to her visit. Dr Hall, the Chief Medical Officer, pointed out that her remit was for hospitals in Turkey only. Nightingale was incensed, but before she could react she collapsed with a Crimean fever. This could have been Crimean-Congo haemorrhagic fever, spread by ticks or human blood with a 20% to 50% mortality, but was more likely to have been brucellosis – from infected milk.

This changed the course of her life. She was delirious for two weeks and when she recovered was too weak to feed herself. Brucellosis would fit with her later problems of neurasthenia (fainting, breathlessness, weakness and inability to digest food), when she rarely left her couch.

On 24 May she was visited by Commander-in-Chief Lord Raglan, who stayed and talked for a long time, and then telegraphed home directly. Four days later Queen Victoria was 'truly thankful to learn that that excellent and valuable person Miss Nightingale is safe'. The Queen sent her a beautiful, specially made brooch. What an impression she had made in only a few short months.

Despite Dr Hall's attempt to put her onto a ship going to England non-stop, she returned to Scutari to convalesce and resume the struggle. There was more opposition and she felt betrayed. By now, however, she had become a legend. At home committees were formed to discuss honouring her – possibly an article of gold or silver, but so much money was donated that a 'Florence Nightingale' fund was set up.

The war came to an end, and just as it did all opposition to her was extinguished by a letter stating: 'Nightingale is recognised by Her Majesty's Government as the General Superintendent of the female nursing establishment of the military hospitals of the army'.

People gradually went home, Dr Hall was given the KCB – 'Knight of the Crimean Burial-grounds,' said Nightingale bitterly.

The last patient was discharged from the Barrack Hospital on 16 July 1856, and Nightingale left for England accompanied by her Aunt Mai on 29 July. She refused the honour of being carried home in a warship, and instead of being met by the massed bands of the army, she took a train and walked home alone from the station.

Acknowledgements

I am grateful to the Florence Nightingale Museum for its help in producing the article.

The address of the museum is: Florence Nightingale Museum, 2 Lambeth Palace Road, London SWI 7EW, Tel: 020 7620 0374. Website: www.florence-nightingale.co.uk

Further reading

Huxley, Elspeth. (1975) *Florence Nightingale*. Weidenfield and Nicholson: London.

Nightingale, Florence. (1859) *Notes on Hospitals*. John W Parker: London

Nightingale, Florence. (1860) *Notes on Nursing – What it is and what it is not*. Harrison: London.

Nightingale, Florence. (1871) *Introductory Notes on Lying-in Institutions*. Longmans. Green and Co.: London.

Woodham Smith, Cecil. (1950) *Florence Nightingale 1820–1910*. Constable: London.

Vicinus Matha and Nergaard, Bea. (1989) *Ever Yours, Florence Nightingale*. Virago Press: London.

Chapter 3
Florence Nightingale part 2: 1856–1910

Introduction

In 1856, an older Florence (see Figure I) once resettled in London after the Crimea, was soon at work trying to improve conditions in the army. Out of the 97,800 British soldiers in the East. 2,700 had been killed, 1,800 died of wounds and 1 7,600 from disease. She kept such a low public profile that many people were unaware she was still alive. However, she had respected Queen Victoria's wish and stayed for a month near Balmoral, seeing the Queen and Prince Albert regularly. They were very supportive of her aims, which included setting up of a Royal Commission (RyC) on 'Regulations affecting the sanitary conditions of the army.' The whole Crimean experience had been exceedingly draining, and indeed by mid-1857 she thought she was dying.

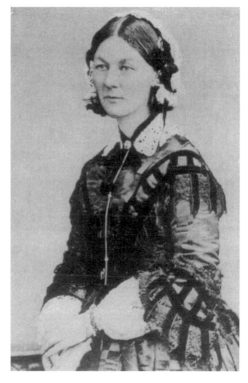

Figure 1   An older Florence Nightingale (Bridgeman Art Library)

She actually lived until she was 90, although for most of the time as an invalid. She toiled incessantly, mainly closeted in a room – at the Burlington Hotel, or later in her house in South Street, Mayfair. She declined a 'grace and favour' apartment in Kensington Palace as being too far removed from the 'centre of things'. South

Street was near the homes of politicians and her rooms faced Hyde Park across the gardens of Grosvenor House. Alas – no more, the whole area was redeveloped into the Grosvenor Hotel and blocks of flats in the 1920s.

She would see visitors by appointment, but often communicated via notes sent down to the hall. She worked through a team of collaborators helpers and mouthpieces, whom she drove forward by her willpower. As time went by famous people came to ask for help. She was visited by Sir John Lawrence before he left to become Viceroy of India (a post she had suggested him for). But as for the Queen of Holland: 'I really feel it is a great honour', wrote Florence. 'She is a Queen of Queens, but it is quite impossible.' She advised the army on hospitals in Canada, and medical services and diet for an expedition to China, and was asked for help by both sides in the Franco-Prussian war.

In order to write her report for the RyC, Florence worked closely with Dr William Farr. He was a pioneer of medical statistics who worked in the Registrar-General's office and was involved with the censuses of 1851 to 1871. Her training in mathematics formed a good basis, and the Crimean experience had underlined the need for accurate figures. She became the 'passionate statistician'. Together they drew up standard lists of diseases, and sets of model statistical forms for hospitals. Her calculations showed that an improvement of the sanitation would lead to a decrease in deaths. Her application of statistics to social dynamics threw up some interesting items: in St Pancreas the civil mortality was 2.2 per 1000. while in the local army barracks it was 10.4. In Kensington, civil mortality was 3.3 per 1000, but in the Knightsbridge barracks it was 17.5. This was despite the fact that the soldiers were young men. and should have been fitter than the general population.

She knew that mortality should be age-related, and that crude death rates could be misleading. Her reports are well provided with accurate tables, and in 1858 she was elected as the first lady member of the Royal Statistical Society (and an honorary member of the American Statistical Association in 1874). The Society held an International Congress in spring 1860, at which 'Miss Nightingale's scheme for uniform hospital statistics' was a major topic. She hosted several breakfasts for members, some of whom were admitted to her bedroom to meet her. Her model data collection forms were well received, and several London hospitals agreed to use them. However, they proved too complicated and were eventually abandoned. A more enduring contribution was her introduction of the 'pictorial chart' or 'coxcomb' for easy presentation of data, which must be the origin of pie charting' (see page 18).

Many people came for advice. One unusual request was for an analysis of resiting St Thomas' Hospital then in the 'Borough' district of London, due to the needs of the railways. Ought the hospital to leave the population it had served for centuries? She complained to Dr Farr that 'the hospital appears to keep its statistics for the purpose of checking obstreperous patients…' Nonetheless she was able to show that by moving it, only a few patients would be disadvantaged.

'It may be a strange principle to enunciate as the first requirement in a hospital that it shall do the sick no harm.' So commences the third edition of *Notes on Hospitals*. The first edition was a reprint of two papers, *The sanitary condition of hospitals,* and *Defects in construction of hospital wards* read for her at a national meeting in 1858, while life at Scutari was still fresh in her mind. 'If the function of the hospital was to kill the sick, comparative mortality figures would be helpful,' she wrote. But she felt that origin and spread of fevers, or the appearance and spread of hospital gangrene, erysipelas and pyaemia are much better tests of the sanitary state of a hospital'. The main problems (drains apart) she felt related to the agglomeration of the sick under one roof, deficiency of space, ventilation and light.

Florence was fairly dismissive of 'contagion' in the *Notes*, indeed she wrote, 'there is no proof of any such thing', and felt that in proper wards patients with 'infectious disease can be nursed together'. However, her Table II (Figure 2) gives mortality figures for hospital staff from 'zymotic' diseases including fever and cholera, in comparison to the female population of London, and her conclusion is that 'hospital hygiene' is important. She later suggested that the ward sister should keep a record of mortality statistics – perhaps the first reference to surveillance of hospital-acquired infections.

TABLE II   Table of the Mortality of Matrons, Sisters, and Nurses, at different Ages, in Fifteen London Hospitals, compared with the Mortality of the Female Population of London.

Ages	Matrons, Sisters, and Nurses (1848–57).		Female Population of London.	
	Annual Rate of Mortality to 1000 living at the respective Ages.			
	By *all* returned Diseases.	By *Zymotic* Diseases.	By *Zymotic* Diseases. (1848–57).	By *all* returned Diseases. (1848–54).
25 to 35	15.89	9.53	2.19	9.92
35–45	15.80	10.94	2.73	14.65
45–55	17.80	11.87	3.17	20.36
55–65	46.36	14.26	4.94	36.02

Figure 2   Florence Nightingale's mortality figures for female staff from 'zymotic' diseases

Her experiences led her to concentrate on the hospital environment rather than the people in it – she was writing before the germ theory of disease, when hospitals were primitive. Lister (1870) also encountered problems in Glasgow in a hospital with the ground floor wards just four feet above the 'cholera' graveyard. His approach was different – to create a clean 'microclimate' on the patient with antiseptics.

The *Notes* continue with other problems: use of absorbent materials for surfaces, defective toilets, furniture, kitchens, laundry, sewerage, inadequate accommodation for nurses, and interestingly enough, construction of hospitals in towns. An appendix describes principles for siting and construction of hospitals based on the 'pure air' principle. They should be outside the town, avoid damp subsoil and sewers, be without cellars, and have pure water. Florence felt this very strongly – why not sell the land in town, which would be valuable, and build in the country, leaving only the accident department and the outpatients in town?

'When fever, erysipelas or gangrene spreads within a hospital, it is no proof of "contagion", but is nature's method of teaching men that her laws are being neglected.' Thus the buildings should be on the 'pavilion' plan – not more than two stories high. Courtyards are to be avoided as reservoirs of stagnant air, as are very tall buildings that might obstruct the light. Kitchens and administrative offices should be sited in a conveniently central position.

Her ward design is shown in Figure 3a, with the dimensions shown in the table (Figure 3b). Non-absorbent walls are specified. together with oiled oak floors. Bedsteads should be of iron with hair mattresses, and furniture of oak. Washing facilities (hot and cold water) are at the ward ends, with outward-flowing sewers. The ward should have no more than 30 beds, and all should be visible from the head nurse's office. Her principles, which were the basis of hospital design for many years, are still very visible in the design of the St Thomas' older buildings – pavilions connected by corridors. They were used for the army hospital at Woolwich (The Royal Herbert Hospital), and indeed still survived in the three identical military hospitals in Malaysia where I worked in the 1960s.

Notes on Nursing – what it is and what it is not was published in December 1859. Although it

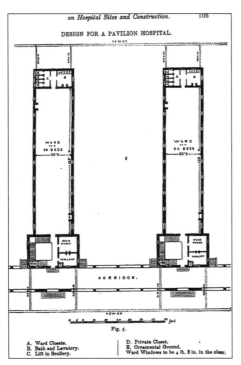

Figure 3a   The 'Nightingale' ward design

	1.		2.	
	Feet.	In.	Feet.	In.
Length of ward	111	6	128	0
Breadth	30	0	30	0
Height	17	0	17	6
Wall spaces between end walls and windows . .	5	0	6	4
Breadth of windows	4	8	4	8
Breath of wall space between windows	9	2	11	4
Height of windows	13	0	13	6
Cubic space per bed	1760	0	2100	0

Figure 3b   Nightingale's dimensions for her ward design (see Figure 3a above)

was not cheap (5/-), 15,000 copies were sold within a month and it became an epoch-making book. 'I am delighted with the *Notes'* wrote a leading surgeon. 'they will do more to call attention to household hygiene (cleanliness, fresh air, sewage disposal) than anything that has ever been written'. It is a delightful book, which also concentrates on the approach to patients, and personal hygiene.

The shadow of the Crimea is not far away. There is a mix of items specific to the 1850s and enduring principles. For example: wearing of crinoline dresses is frowned on, 'the fidget of silk and of crinoline… will do a patient more harm than all the medicines in the world will do him good. Fortunate it is, if her skirts do not catch fire and if the nurse does not give herself up as a sacrifice together with the patient – to be burnt in her own petticoats'.

Other instructions are surprisingly up with the times, particularly the advice on handwashing. Florence may not have known about germs, but she writes: 'Every nurse ought to be careful to wash her hands frequently during the day.' She continues: 'By simply washing or sponging with water, you do not really clean your skin. Take a rough towel, dip one corner in very hot water – if a little spirit be added – it will be more effective, and then rub as if you were rubbing the towel into your skin with your fingers.'

In conclusion, she emphasises the duty of prevention for the surgical nurse to beware of fever, hospital gangrene or pyaemia. She must ever be 'on guard against want of cleanliness, foul air, want of light and warmth'.

Florence soon became immersed in other things, including St Thomas' and the nurse training school. A lesser known outcome of the Nightingale fund was the establishment of a school for midwives in the 'new' part of King's College Hospital in 1862. However, after six years, the management committee noted that there had been an unacceptable mortality of 33.3 mothers per 1000 from childbirth fever. The worst year followed admission of a lady with erysipelas, who later died. The result was that the wards were shut down, and Florence was stimulated to study the problem of why it was dangerous to give birth in hospitals.

Notes on Lying-in Institutions was the result. Tables of statistics from across Europe are everywhere, together with analyses of hospital design. She uses some of the same statistics as Semmelweis (his book came out in 1864, but is not mentioned). As for Vienna – she accepted the idea of the medical students as the cause of the problem, although she notes without comment that the death rate dropped after 1847, and indeed in September 1856 (when Semmelweis's handwashing was underway), there were more deaths in the midwives clinic (105) than in the students' (13). Sadly, although she mentions Skoda and Rokitansky by name (Semmelweis's teachers), they are only quoted as supporters of contagion, foul air and miasmas. However, she notes with disfavour that the postmortem room windows at King's were next to the postnatal ward.

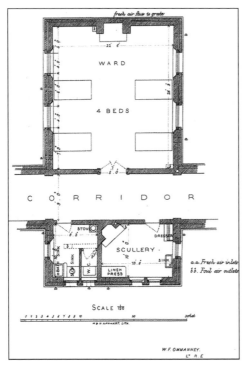

Figure 4   The plan for maternity hospitals

The positive outcome was a plan for maternity hospitals, still based on the pavilion system, but with only four beds per unit, and a scullery and bathroom across the corridor (see Figure 4). This had already been tried out with success (as far as maternal deaths went) in some military hospitals. In the plan, she allows for a 'segregation ward'. 'A ward is unfortunately necessary, completely isolated, where a sick case, brought in with smallpox or erysipelas could be delivered entirely separately, or where a case of puerperal fever or peritonitis (which should never arise in a properly constructed and managed institution) could be transferred. If puerperal fever should occur, no new admissions should be allowed until the buildings have been thoroughly cleansed, lime-washed and aired. The segregation ward... must have its own sink.'

Thus even though Florence did not know about bacteria and was dismissive of contagion when she wrote these books, she nonetheless stated many of the principles of infection control. How much she later accepted the germ theory is a topic for discussion (see: www.florence-nightingale-avenging-angel.co.uk).

She lived another 39 years, mainly in her house in South Street, but moved to look after her parents in their old age. In 1857, she had met a 56-year-old widower Sir Henry Verney owner of Claydon House near Buckingham. He fell in love with her, but received the usual refusal. He married Parthe. Florence always remained a friend, and later looked after her sister in her final illness. She was a frequent visitor to Claydon House, which is now a National Trust property. In it, there is a museum containing many memorabilia – in particular pictures of the Crimea, a lovely display on the owl, a reconstruction of Florence's bedroom, and an orange given to her in the Crimea.

She died in 1910 and in accordance with her wishes was buried not in Westminster Abbey, but in the family grave at East Wellow. in the New Forest (see Figure 5). She was however carried to her grave by six sergeants from the British Army.

In contrast to the other pioneers in this series memorabilia are readily available. The Nightingale Museum in London is well worth a visit, as is Claydon House, and the lovely church at East Wellow. Her medals are in the National Army Museum in Chelsea, together with some jewellery and an original lamp. Statues of Sidney Herbert, Florence and the Crimea Memorial – said to contain metal from Russian guns – stand in London's Waterloo Place and face St James's Park. This is a fitting place to end my story about this exceptional lady, aware that I have only skimmed selectively over the surface of her life.

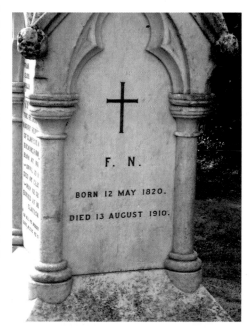

Figure 5   Florence was buried in the family grave at East Wellow (Newsom)

Acknowledgements

I am grateful to the Florence Nightingale Museum for its help in producing the article.

The address of the museum is: Florence Nightingale Museum, 2 Lambeth Palace Road. London SW1 7EW. Tel: 020 7620 0374, See:website: www.florence-nightingale.co.uk

Further reading
Lister J. (1870) On the effects of the antiseptic system of treatment upon the salubrity of a surgical hospital. *Lancet* (i): 40.

Nightingale F. (1859) *Notes on Hospitals.* John W Parker: London.

Nightingale F. (1860) *Notes on Nursing – what it is and what it is not.* Harrison: London.

Nightingale F. (1871) *Introductory Notes on Lying-in Institutions.* Longmans. Green and Company: London.

Small H. (2000) *Florence Nightingale. Avenging Angel.* Isis: Oxford.

Vicinus M, Nergaard B. (1989) *Ever Yours. Florence Nightingale.* Virago Press: London.

Woodham Smith C. (1950) *Florence Nightingale 1820–1910.* Constable: London.

Chapter 4

Joseph Lister and safe surgery

Introduction

Joseph Lister (see Figure 1) equals Ignaz Philip Semmelweis as a major innovator in infection control. He laid the foundations for modern surgery through his introduction of the 'antiseptic barrier' technique, which was the predecessor of the current 'aseptic' surgery. He is rightly called one of the great benefactors of mankind.

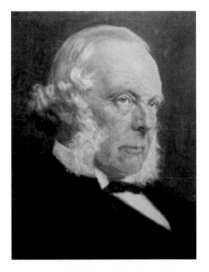

The lives of the two men have interesting similarities and contrasts. Both came from well-off families, capable of supporting them in their education. Lister was born in 1827, so was ten years younger and lived throughout in a peaceful Britain, unlike Semmelweis who encountered revolution and war in Austro-Hungary. Semmelweis was a collector of epidemiological data, and made his discovery in 1848 while a young doctor in training – and was effectively sacked as a result. He did not publish his results until 1861.

Lister, on the other hand, was a 'hands-on' experimenter, encouraged by his father who gave him an excellent

Figure 1   Joseph Lister (1827–1912) (Royal College of Surgeons of England)

microscope (see page 58) while he was still a student. He was already a professor when he made his great contribution, which was in 1865 the year of Semmelweis's death. He published the results in the *British Medical Journal* in 1867.

The two never met, and Lister was unaware of Semmelweis's work until late in life. He did, however, meet the great Viennese pathologist Rokitansky (who taught Semmelweis) when Rokitansky visited Lister's father in 1842, and again on his honeymoon visit to Vienna in 1856. Although Lister's father, a strict

Quaker, was in the wine trade, like many other Victorians he was an 'amateur' scientist. He had invented the 'achromatic' lens, which he ground himself, hence coming to the notice of Rokitansky. He was a Fellow of the Royal Society, of which his son was to become President.

Lister's first publications were made while he was still a student at University College Hospital, and must have reflected his father's interest as they reported microscopic studies on the iris and on the contractile elements in skin responsible for 'goose pimples'. In 1853, having obtained his Fellowship of the Royal College of Surgeons, his teachers suggested he visit Professor Syme in Edinburgh (the most famous surgeon of the time – still remembered in Syme's amputation) and then go to the continent before settling down to a career in London. In the event he never got beyond Edinburgh, where he became Syme's assistant, and later married his daughter Agnes.

His surgery and teaching both developed to such an extent that seven years later at the early age of 33 he became the Regius Professor of Surgery to Glasgow University, where he settled down to do his research and develop his 'antiseptic principle'.

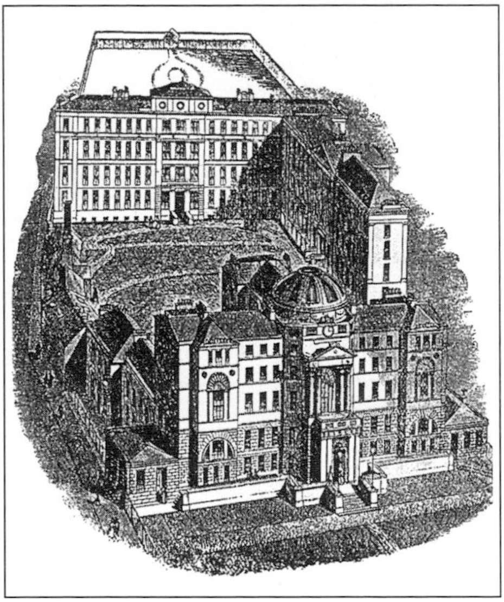

Figure 2   At the time of Lister's investigations into antiseptic surgery The Glasgow Royal Infirmary was a large and well-equipped hospital, but gangrene was rampant

Historical context

Up until this time surgery had mainly been that of trauma. The most expert surgeons were military men who were able to remove a limb at speed. Most wounds became infected and the presence of pus was looked on as 'laudable', in that it showed the body was responding to the infection.

After even a simple operation the surgeon was likened to a husbandmen, who having sown his field, waits with resignation for what the harvest may bring and reaps it, fully conscious of his own impotence against the elemental powers that may pour down rain hurricane and hailstorm. Well endowed and built hospitals like the Glasgow Royal Infirmary (see Figure 2) were quite common.

However, Sir James Young Simpson, the obstetrician from Edinburgh (of whom we will hear more), said (in 1861): 'The man laid on the operating table of one of our surgical hospitals is exposed to more chances of death than the English soldier on the field of Waterloo.' As late as 1874 Sir John Erichsen, the top London surgeon (for whom Lister did his first house job) suggested that hospitals should periodically be razed to the ground and rebuilt to combat the 'hospital gangrene'.

Not all was doom and gloom. The aforementioned James Simpson had invented the use of chloroform as an anaesthetic, allowing operations to become pain-free. Like Semmelweis, Lister regarded the wounds as undergoing 'putrefaction'. When discussing this with his colleagues, he was recommended to read the writings of Pasteur, who had just published his work disproving the theory of 'spontaneous generation'.

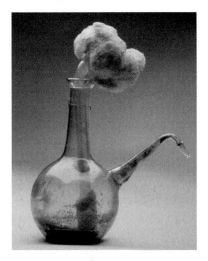

Pasteur used 'Swan-necked' flasks (see Figure 3) filled with a yeast extract, which he boiled. Then he sealed the neck of each flask and as the liquid cooled a small vacuum was created. The flasks were then opened in different locations to allow air to enter, and resealed. The sites used to open the flasks varied from a Paris room full of dusty air, to Mont Blanc. Growth only occurred in the flasks opened in dirty conditions. Later he showed that even in these, a flask could remain open to the air and not become infected as long as it had a convoluted neck capable of preventing the dust in the air from reaching the fluid.

Figure 3   Lister's version of the 'Swan necked flask' (Royal College of Surgeons of England)

'It (the fluid) is dumb,' he said, 'because I have kept from it the only thing that man cannot produce, from the germs which float in the air.'

Pasteur wrote: 'In the field of observation, chance favours the mind which is already prepared.' Lister realised that 'the germs that float in the air', and probably were found on hands, instruments and ligatures, caused the putrefaction of wounds. Later he repeated Pasteur's experiments and made many bacterial cultures to prove the point. If he could put a barrier between his patient's wound and the germs, all should be well. There remained one way – to apply some chemical in such a manner that not only would the microbes already present be destroyed, but also the germ-killing substance must act as a barrier between the wound and all sources of outside infection, so that the entrance of further microbes would be prevented (Lister's own description of his 'Antiseptic System').

What to use? Clearly he could not use heat. He tried various substances without success. Then one day he noted in the newspaper that carbolic acid had been used to good effect in treating the sewage of Carlisle. He obtained a sample of 'German creosote' from a colleague. This was the crude product (as applied to the garden fence !). It had a foul smell, and was immiscible with water, but did mix with oil.

Pioneering treatment

The first patient to be successfully treated with the new system was James Greenlees, a frightened 11-year-old boy, with a compound fracture of the left leg from having been run over by a cart. He had a wound about 1.5 inches long over the fracture.

The treatment consisted of an application of undiluted carbolic to all parts of the wound, which was then covered with lint or calico soaked in carbolic. To lessen the evaporation, this was covered with a sheet of tin or lead, which had been already sterilised by immersion in the carbolic. Four days later when the wound was examined, there was a singular absence of the usual signs of inflammation, just a slight blush on the adjacent skin. The dressing was renewed using carbolic diluted in water. Five days later the wound was satisfactory and the dressing was changed to one impregnated with the carbolic acid diluted in 20 parts of olive oil. Six weeks after admission, James had a united fracture and a healed wound – an unheard of event.

Lister's second patient had a similar course to begin with, but unfortunately Lister had to leave town for some weeks. A small sore that he left with healthy granulations became infected and the patient died. But ten more cases of compound fracture were treated and eight recovered.

Lister had learnt that carbolic would do the job. It had an anaesthetic action, so was painless, and when mixed with blood in the wound formed a hard crust, able to prevent ingress of pathogens. However, it was a strong irritant. Fortunately by now he had obtained a supply of much purer carbolic acid from a chemist in Manchester. This was a crystalline powder, soluble in 20 parts of water and readily soluble in oil. A strong solution boiled in linseed oil was very effective, but much less irritant. Different application methods were tried: lint was replaced by a putty made of carbonate of lime mixed with carbolic oil spread over tinfoil.

Peer criticism

Now it was time to broadcast his results, which he did at scientific meetings (notably in Dublin), and then by short reports in the *Lancet,* followed by the paper in the *British Medical Journal.*

Unfortunately all his first patients had compound fractures, and so could have been expected to have infected wounds. His 'principles' were thus regarded purely as an 'antiseptic treatment', which had been known about for years.

Simpson spoke disparagingly about them at the Dublin meeting, and was thought to be the author of a scurrilous article in an Edinburgh daily newspaper a few weeks later. He said that the continental surgeons had been doing this for years. The *Lancet* then entered the fray, publishing among other criticisms one from Simpson accusing Lister of ignorance. Lister was very cross to have been made to appear in such an unfavourable light, so that his invaluable work was set back at the start.

However, he persisted in Glasgow and had much to reassure him. Although the surgical wing of the infirmary was new, with good ventilation and well-spaced beds, hospital gangrene was rampant, except in Lister's emergency ward. The mortality was so great in the other emergency ward (only 12 feet across the passage) that it had to be closed for an inspection of the drains and foundations. This revealed an unexpected horror – namely that on a level with the floors of both emergency wards, separated by an area only four foot wide, were the upper-most coffins of a mass grave used for the victims of the 1849 cholera epidemic. A Glasgow newspaper reported that at least 5,000 other bodies were also to be found in mass paupers' pits all around the infirmary, which in any case backed onto a churchyard. However, in Lister's ward not one case of hospital gangrene, pyaemia or erysipelas occurred.

The next major event occurred two years later in 1869, when he was invited back to replace Syme as the Professor in Edinburgh. Simpson had disappeared from the scene, so he had a warm welcome, and was pleased to be back. Agnes was delighted when they moved into the Syme's house in Charlotte Square. She was a perfect partner for Lister, being both technician and secretary as well as much-loved wife. The house became one of the world's first bacteriology laboratories when Lister decided to study lactic fermentation in the front room. He originally used 'boiled' liqueur glasses covered with a glass cap, then later a stand with small tubes. With this he was the first person ever to grow bacteria in pure culture albeit in liquid. He also grew *penicillium* and noted that it produced volatile products and a smell, but did not go any further – or he might have added the discovery of penicillin to his achievements. He was more interested in microbes as a whole, and did not relate particular germs to human disease.

The 'antiseptic method' was refined and extended. In 1870 he became Surgeon-in Ordinary (Scotland) to Queen Victoria: no sinecure as he had an abscess to drain. On this occasion he inserted a rubber tube (previously soaked in carbolic) into the Queen's abscess. The drain, the first ever to be used, worked perfectly. Lister also pioneered the use of catgut.

The next major change to the antiseptic technique was the introduction of the carbolic acid spray during operations, in order to destroy the bacteria in the air. The original sprays were cumbersome, and the 'donkey engine' – so called because it required relays of students to keep pumping it – sat on a large tripod. Later a smaller steam-operated instrument was used. My vision of the Lister operation is indeed one with the latter spray in use as shown in Figure 4, which shows an operation being performed in 1880 in Aberdeen.

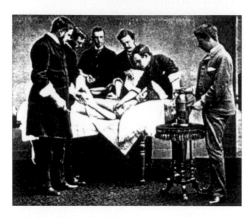

Figure 4   A 'Listerian' operation, at Aberdeen. Fourth from the left is Alexander Ogston (Department of Surgery, Aberdeen University)

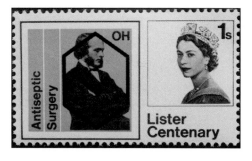

Figure 5   Lister's work was recognised on a special set of stamps

The message spread slowly, with continental surgeons being the most enthusiastic to adopt the methods, which is perhaps a reflection of the political ties with Scotland. Later the technique was used in the English provinces, but not in London.

However, the spray must have been a problem to the operators. Although it may be thought to be Lister's trademark, and indeed appeared on the second of the centenary postage stamps (see Figure 5), it was in fact a needless complication. The German enthusiastic supporters of Lister said 'Away with the spray'. Eventually Lister conceded it was not required, saying: 'I feel ashamed that I should have ever recommended it for destroying microbes in the air,' but adding: 'If we were to give up all washing and irrigation of the wound, our vigilance must be redoubled.'

In 1887, aged 50, he returned to London, as the Professor of Surgery at King's College Hospital. Here he set about converting the surgeons to his system. It was a painfully slow business, but helped by his dignified and charming personality. By now he was a much-revered figure. He was created Baron Lister in 1883, made a Peer in 1897, and was one of the first 12 people to be awarded the Order of Merit by King Edward VIIth.

He also had a major role in International Science. He maintained good relations with Louis Pasteur, and had the satisfaction of bringing him together with Koch at an International Congress in London. He represented the Royal Society at Pasteur's 70th birthday celebrations where, to his embarrassment, after he spoke of the debt surgery owed to Pasteur, the latter threw his arms around him and kissed him on both cheeks – to the thunderous applause of an audience of 2500.

Lister lived to a ripe old age, although sadly his wife died in 1893, while he lived on until 1912. Although he had been one of the most successful doctors that ever lived, in his old age, like Semmelweis, he dwelt on the controversy surrounding his early work, and feared he had been misunderstood. In contrast however, his work was widely acclaimed during his lifetime.

'*Mankind looks grateful now on thee For what thou didst in* surgery. And death must often go amiss by smelling antiseptic *bliss.*' (Prof Stromeyer, Hanover).

Acknowledgements

I am grateful to the Royal College of Surgeons for Figures 1 and 3, and the Department of Surgery, Aberdeen University for Figure 4.

Further reading

Godlee RJ. *Lord Lister.* London, Macmillan and Co, 1917. (This is the 'official' biography written by Lister's nephew. Interestingly enough his great granddaughter is Fiona Godlee, now editor of the British Medical Journal).

Watson Cheyne W. *Lister and his achievement.* London, Longman's Green and co, 1925. (Watson Cheyne was Lister's Assistant, who followed him from Edinburgh to London, and translated Koch's work into English).

Guthrie D. *Lord Lister.* Edinburgh, E&S Livingstone, 1949. (A much more readable and smaller book!).

[Copies of all three books are to be found on abebooks.com – usually for under £20.00]

Newsom SWB. Pioneers in infection control – Joseph Lister. *Journal of Hospital Infection,* 2003, **55**: 246–253.

Chapter 5

Pasteur, the lynch-pin

Introduction

Louis Pasteur in many ways is best considered as the 'lynch-pin', whose work tied together that of the other pioneers. He was born in 1822, four years after Semmelweis and in the same decade as Lister.

Unlike the others mentioned in this series he was never medically qualified. True to form he had controversies with Robert Koch, but was greatly admired by Joseph Lister.

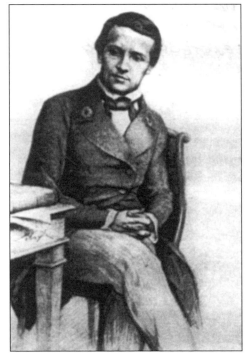

Figure 1   Louis Pasteur (1822–1895)

Early years

Pasteur had a strong family background – his father had been a sergeant in Napoleon's armies, and retired to run a tannery in Arbois, a town well to the east of Paris – in fact near to Switzerland. He passionately desired the best for Louis, and did his best to send him to a good school where the academic life could take hold.

Louis's one aim was to be taken on at the École Normale Superior, a highly competitive national school in Paris that Napoleon had founded for training young professors. Implicit in becoming a student was the duty to work for ten years as a 'public instructor', i.e. a state servant.

An early trip to Paris (when aged 15) to prepare for the exams was soon aborted – Pasteur felt very homesick, and his father couldn't bear to lose him and came (unannounced) to take him home.

By the time Pasteur was 20 he had passed the entrance exam, but only in 16th place. This was not good enough for a perfectionist, so he took it again a year later, and honour was satisfied when he came fifth.

Discovering science

What type of student would he become? At school he was good at art – and did fine portraits of his family.

However, fired up by lectures from Professor Dumas at the Sorbonne, he abandoned this in favour of science, to which from then on – apart from family matters and holidays (usually back in Arbois) – he devoted his whole life, ensuring that wherever he was he had a laboratory to hand.

He described the lectures in a letter home: 'you cannot imagine what a crowd of people come to these lectures. The room is immense and always full, we have to arrive half an hour early to get a good seat, and there is always a great deal of applause.'

The eager student arrived a week early to the École Normale, and was often to be found in the library, despite his father's warnings of 'do not work too much'. A topic much in vogue at the school was that of crystals and their optical properties.

After listening to a lecture from a Professor Biot, Pasteur took it upon himself to study crystals of tartaric acid (found during the fermentation of wine – so of interest to the French). He had to grow his own crystals, study their shapes and make his own polarimeter to study their effect on light. Even with such simple equipment, he was able to define left and right polarising crystals and the inactive 'racemic' mixture of both.

Once he had confirmed his experiments he was so excited he ran into the laboratory hall, gave the first person he met (a laboratory technician) a hug, and said: 'I am so happy, I have just made a great discovery, but I am shaking all over and unable to set my eyes again to the polarimeter.'

Building a reputation

Professor Biot heard of his work and sent for the young student, and asked him to repeat his experiments, finishing them off for himself. Having satisfied himself of the truth, Biot was moved to take Pasteur's arm and say: 'My dear boy, I have loved science so much during my life, that this touches my very heart.'

This was an excellent start for the 25-year-old student – addressed by the 70-year-old top scientist. At a stroke Pasteur had established his reputation.

Moving on

Pasteur's career was then interrupted by the Minister of Public Instruction – it was time for him to go to Dijon as professor of physics. There was nothing Biot or the others could do, although he was allowed to stay in Paris until November and finish some work suggested by Biot, who 'thought and dreamt of nothing but these new investigations'.

Pasteur's friends and collaborators desperately wanted him back, and he wrote to the Minister hoping for a return. The result was a new post at Strasbourg. Here at least was a good university, and the Rector was very welcoming with invitations to his house.

Pasteur could feel the happiness within, so much so that only a fortnight later he wrote to Laurent (the Rector): 'An offer of the greatest importance to me and your family is about to be made to you on my behalf (by his father). I have absolutely no fortune: my only means are good health, some courage, and my position in the University.' To Marie Laurent he wrote later: 'I, who did so love my crystals…'

Actually he got both. His wife was an amazing person, running the family, providing stability, encouraging his science and even acting as his secretary on occasion, like Agnes Lister.

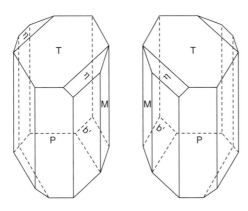

Figure 2   Pasteur's early work was on crystals

Five years later, the Minister made him dean of a new faculty of sciences in Lille, another major move (and there was no Eurostar in those days!).

This provided a better income and more scope for continuing researches, still mainly aimed at crystals, but by now biology in the shape of their interaction with fungi had taken a hold on him, together with the idea that optically active compounds were associated with living organisms.

At Lille he was expected to be of practical use, as well as teaching chemistry. A local industrialist came for help when his production of alcohol from beetroot failed. Pasteur noted that yeasts (previously thought to be just catalysts) normally found in the fermenting beetroot were associated with other small bodies. Fermentation required yeasts, but the other bodies were like those in the 'lactic ferment', which turned milk sour.

Life became more complex when he returned after only three years in Lille as administrator to the École Normale, which he felt was 'only a shadow of its former self'.

Debunking the myth of spontaneous generation

Research continued, however, and he became convinced that 'spontaneous generation' of life was a myth. The yeasts did not just appear in the beetroot juice. One simple test he did was to remove the juice from an undamaged grape through a needle and show that provided it was kept away from contamination it did not ferment.

By the age of 40 he had demonstrated that fermentations were due to micro-organisms, and that to study fermentation you needed to prepare the correct sterile culture medium, then add a trace of the pure ferment. He had thus laid the foundations of microbiology.

The next 15 years' research was spent enlarging his views on microbes, and helping to solve a series of very practical problems. In my previous chapter on Lister I noted the use of Swan-necked flasks containing a boiled culture medium, which remained sterile unless exposed to contaminated air.

Pasteur himself used his summer holidays to go climbing in the Alps to open flasks in the clean air – he would have liked to go up in a balloon, but this was impossible – so he had to climb up himself and open the flasks on a glacier. As Pasteur had predicted, the liquid in these flasks remained sterile despite exposure to the mountain air, unlike those that had been opened in a Paris street. With

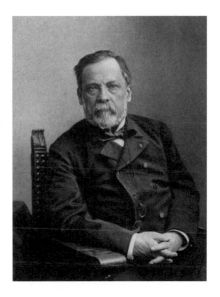

Figure 3   Pasteur's work was revolutionary in discovering the link between bacteria and disease

such tests he effectively demolished the theory of spontaneous generation.

By now he was a well-recognised scientist, and in 1862 (sadly just after Biot's death) he was elected to the prestigious Academy of Sciences. Napoleon asked to meet him, and took a continuing interest in his work.

Arbois has been a centre of wine production since Roman days, although today we rarely hear of Jura wines. A special type of wine was made from grapes laid out to dry on straw – so it is no great surprise that Pasteur's childhood friends (now vineyard owners) complained when acidity ruined their wines.

Family summer holidays were spent with the grandparents in Arbois, and so Pasteur had time for investigating the problem. Like the beetroot one, he put it down to 'parasitic vegetations' (bacteria) and showed that if you heated the wine to 50°C to 60°C, these were then killed, but the wine quality was maintained. Interestingly enough, this method was only later applied to milk, which even today is 'pasteurised' to prevent the 'lactic fermentation'.

Another French industry in seemingly terminal decline by 1865 was that of silkworm cultivation. The silkworms were dying for unknown reasons. Dumas, his old chemistry teacher – now a Senator and agriculture minister, wrote to plead with Pasteur to go and sort it out.

The old teacher/pupil ties were great, so Pasteur agreed to go, though not without some misgiving, for as he wrote: 'Remember if you please that I have never even touched a silkworm.'

He set off for the Cevennes, but had only been away ten days before news of his father's terminal illness reached him. By the time he got to Arbois, Pasteur senior was dead. Soon afterwards one of his daughters died, and a second died of typhoid the following year.

However, work on silkworms continued. In 1867 he requested some more laboratory facilities from Napoleon. These were immediately granted. He eventually showed that two distinct diseases were involved, one nutritional and the other caused by a protozoon, and that by careful application of hygienic measures the latter could be avoided.

Thus by 1870 Pasteur had one 'infection controlled' accolade, although silkworms were hardly of interest to doctors – despite the fact that the basic control measures were those used today in hospitals.

In 1867 Pasteur gave up his administrative role at the École Normale and was appointed Professor of Chemistry to the Sorbonne. By now many international prizes and medals were his.

However, in 1868 he had a stroke. He had woken that October day with a strange tingling in one hand, but insisted on going to the library. His wife must have had a presentiment, as she went with him.

However, all was well till bedtime when he became dizzy and unable to speak. His speech recovered a few days later – 'mind active', wrote his doctor, 'would willingly talk science'. Three months later back in the Cevennes he was directing silkworm investigations from his couch.

Medical breakthroughs

When will I get to the point, you may ask. Not until 1877 did Pasteur turn his attention to medicine. Lister by then had perfected his 'antiseptic system', based on Pasteur's work, to control and prevent infections in wounds (which could not be pasteurised). He had also succeeded in preparing pure cultures of bacteria in liquid media.

Lister always acknowledged his debt to Pasteur, and wrote to him in 1874: 'I need hardly add that it would afford me the greatest gratification to show you how greatly surgery is indebted to you.'

Anthrax and chicken cholera

Even then it was veterinary medicine that first caught Pasteur's attention, through the disease of sheep called 'splenic fever' that killed 20% to 50% of some flocks. This turned out to be anthrax, which had already been attributed to bacteria by Koch's work some years earlier.

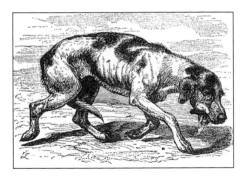

Figure 4   Pasteur developed a vaccination for rabies which helped secure his place in history (Wellcome Images)

Next, Pasteur turned to the cause of chicken cholera. In both cases he isolated the bacteria, then noted that on laboratory culture the chicken cholera bacteria changed so they lost their virulence. In the case of the anthrax bacteria, culture at 42°C or 43°C was enough to render them harmless.

So on 5 May 1879 a famous assembly of scientists – mainly sceptics – assembled at a farm at Pouilly-le-Fort to see Pasteur infect sheep and cows with his 'attenuated' anthrax bacteria. He was well aware, as he lectured to his visitors, that most of them expected the animals to die.

On 31 May everyone was back at the farm to watch a vet inoculate the animals with fully virulent bacteria. 'Make sure you shake the cultures well first', said one sceptic, 'the nastier germs will be at the bottom'. The bottles were shaken very vigorously, and the vet proceeded to give the animals three times the normal lethal dose.

The next few days were ones of anguish – several of the vaccinated animals developed a fever, and one sheep looked on the verge of death – but on the next morning all the vaccinated animals were well. All the unvaccinated animals died, and the experiment was deemed a stunning success.

Robert Koch

Enter Koch and controversy. Koch had attempted vaccine production by growing the bacilli at 42°C by a different method (on agar rather than in a liquid), and failed – the bacteria were still virulent. Pasteur meanwhile arranged for some tests of his vaccine in Germany and, possibly to Koch's annoyance, German farmers began to clamour for it.

When an international congress was held in Geneva in 1882, Koch (now buoyed up by his successful work on tuberculosis) got up after a paper by Pasteur and said how disappointed he was in that he had hoped to hear something new. 'As I don't speak French well and Pasteur cannot speak German', he continued, 'I will continue our discussion in the journals.'

Pasteur replied that he had presented new material and would await publication of Koch's comments. To his assistant he wrote: 'Koch acted ridiculous and made a fool of himself.'

By 1888 Pasteur was head of a purpose-built institute in Paris in which many of the basic discoveries of infectious diseases and of immunology were made, and indeed continue to be so (for example Luc Montagnier, now a Nobel prize winner, discoverer of HIV).

Rabies

However, Pasteur's last big work was, in many ways, the most amazing. He developed a vaccine for an infection without being able to isolate or grow any bacteria – namely rabies, which is of course caused by a virus.

At the time, rabies was a terrifying and mystical disease. Renée Dubos, a famous bacteriologist of later years noted that 'although the Pouilly-le-Fort experiment had captured the public interest, it was the prophylaxis of rabies that made microbiological science an established religion and surrounded its creator with the halo of sainthood.'

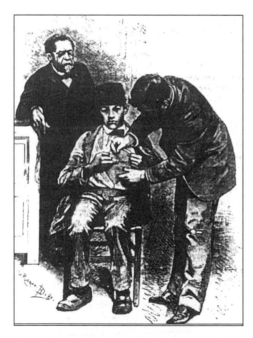

Figure 5   Joseph Meister was the first of many children and adults to be vaccinated against rabies (from an old French magazine)

Rabies (Latin for madness) is an acute infection caused by a virus and transmitted by the saliva of an infected animal (Figure 4). Pasteur demonstrated that the infective agent, called a virus (Latin for poison), was present in the spinal cord of infected animals.

Bearing in mind his ability to make 'attenuated' bacteria into vaccines – he tried growing the virus in rabbits. By injecting a rabbit with material from the dog's spinal cord, he found that the virus changed – the rabbit died, and on removing the spinal cord and placing it into another rabbit, the virus became more poisonous for the rabbit. The incubation period of the disease became shorter and shorter as the material was 'passaged' through successive rabbits. However, the material became less dangerous to the dog.

Pasteur then went one stage further and removed the spinal cord of a dead rabbit and dried it for 14 days, by which time it could no longer cause the disease in dogs.

The next step was to see how immunised dogs reacted to a challenge dose of fresh material from a dog just died of rabies. Not every dog was protected and there were some 'accidents', to use Pasteur's own words, but by 6 July 1885 he had data on 50 dogs – all of which had been protected.

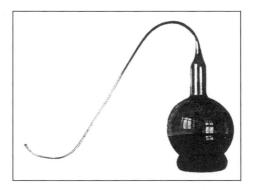

Figure 6   Pasteur used Swan-necked flasks to disprove the theory of spontaneous generation of bacteria

On this day a nine-year-old boy, Joseph Meister, was brought into his laboratory after having been bitten severely on the hands and leg by a rabid dog. Two medical consultants were called in and both agreed that the wounds would be fatal.

The vaccine was administered and on 26 October Pasteur was able to announce to the Academie of Sciences that Joseph was well. It was indeed a fittingly triumphant end to Pasteur's career. Within 15 months of Joseph's injections, no fewer than 2490 people had received the vaccine, and Pasteur had the great satisfaction of seeing the ready acceptance of his work.

Joseph Meister became the gatekeeper to the Pasteur Institute. In 1940, 55 years later, he committed suicide rather than open Pasteur's burial crypt to German soldiers.

Professional recognition

On 27 December 1892, the great hall of the Sorbonne was filled with scientists assembled to celebrate Pasteur's 70th birthday. He entered leaning on the arm of the President of the Republic. Many eulogies were spoken, and Lister rose to embrace Pasteur.

The sight of the two men gave the impression of a brotherhood of science labouring to diminish the sorrows of humanity. Lister deserves the last word: 'you have,' he said, raised the veil which for centuries had covered the infectious diseases: you have discovered and demonstrated their microbian nature.'

Further reading

Dubos R. *Pasteur and modern science*. Washington, American Society for Microbiology: 1998. (Modern paberback reprint of 1960's classic).

Cuny H. *Louis Pasteur – The Man and his theories*. London, Souvenir Press, 1965.

Chapter 6

Robert Koch, father of medical microbiology part 1: 1843–1890

Introduction

In the bacteriology lab the staff are always talking about Gram's stain and Petri dishes. These are basic everyday tools. Both were minor modifications of Koch's techniques.

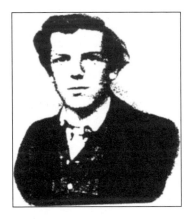

Figure 1   Robert Koch (1843–1910)
(Thomas Brock)

Actually Gram (page 64) developed his stain during a one-month research project and never thought about it again, while Petri, although head of a sanatorium, was an imposter who often appeared in the uniform of a military doctor, but was not medically qualified at all.

Sadly, we rarely, if ever, refer to Robert Koch (see Figure 1), although he was the founder of medical microbiology, and one of the pioneers of heat sterilisation. Unlike the others, however. his work resulted in the award of a Nobel prize.

Studious and hard working from an early age

Koch was born in Germany, not far from Hanover in 1843, around the time when Semmelweis was collecting his data. Like Semmelweis and Lister he came from a middle-class background but was one of a family of 13, 11 of whom lived to adult life, so there could not have been much money to spare.

He was a very intelligent child. He was much influenced by his uncle Edward, who was devoted to nature study photography (at a time when to obtain a photograph was a triumph).

At school he excelled in mathematics and science, but tried hard at learning English and French, an indicator perhaps of his aim to travel.

By the time he came to leave school he had a solid girlfriend called Emmy. So he turned down the idea of emigrating to the US and becoming successful in business like his two elder brothers, and went to Gottingen University to study medicine.

He published two papers while still a student, thanks to stimulation from some excellent teachers. He qualified in 1866 and married Emmy in 1867.

From medical assistant in Hamburg to amateur researcher as a country GP

Marriage meant getting a job, and quickly too; he gave up romantic ideas of being a ship's doctor, and went to the Hamburg General Hospital as a medical assistant. However, although he enjoyed the job and was able to do some research, it was obvious he would never earn enough money to support a family. So he moved nearer home and worked in a village where he could combine a none too exciting job working with retarded children with that of the village GP.

Country life allowed plenty of time for nature study, Emmy was a great help in collecting samples of plants, pond water etc. for Robert to examine with his microscope. However, finance – budgets were a problem even in 1868 – forced them to move.

After a certain amount of trial and error (the population of Niemegk preferred faith healers to doctors!), he got a government job as a 'District Health Officer' in Wollstein, a small town far away from home in eastern Germany. When he arrived he was an enthusiastic 29-year-old amateur scientist, when he left eight years later he was well on his way to winning the Nobel prize.

Anthrax studies

How did this happen? Well, he soon built up a successful medical practice, and then with his enthusiasm and his wife's support part of his examination room was curtained off as a laboratory. Careful budgeting allowed the purchase of a better microscope, which he set up to take photographs (see Figure 2).

His first foray into bacteriology concerned anthrax. This was mainly an epidemic disease of sheep and cattle, usually fatal, with occasional human cases. Anthrax bacilli form heat resistant spores. The disease is rare today, but the germs are still of interest – recent events have shown their application as a form of germ warfare.

By chance, on 23 December 1875, Koch was asked to examine an animal thought to have died of anthrax. His microscope revealed many bacteria in the animal's blood, which he then inoculated onto a rabbit's ear.

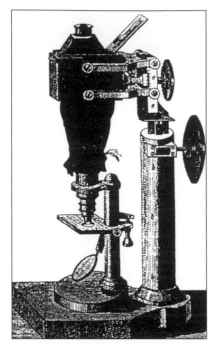

Figure 2   Abbe's design and Zeiss development of the oil-immersion lens revolutionised microbial microscopy (Thomas Brock)

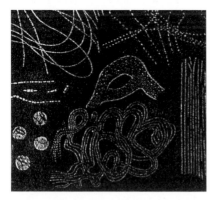

Figure 3   Anthrax bacilli photographed by Robert Koch

The animal died on Christmas Eve, and so Koch removed its ear and put it into alcohol. Then, on Christmas Day. he examined it with the microscope. It was full of the same bacteria, so he took some tissue from the dead rabbit and introduced it into the eye of a second rabbit. This too died, and turbidity in its eye was due to multiplication of the bacteria in the aqueous humour.

This gave Koch the idea of using corneal fluid to grow bacteria. Thus in one short week he had performed microscopy, animal experiments and bacterial culture – all successfully.

The anthrax bacilli that he saw (see Figure 3) are unique in their ability to form 'ropes'. The spores are highly resistant and indeed Gruinard, a small island off Scotland, was rendered uninhabitable by some anthrax 'germ warfare' tests during the second world war.

Close to home, a field in Cambridge was known to contain the grave of a horse that died of anthrax in the 1930s, but even as late as 1980, it was left alone, although surrounded by housing estates.

First contact with Professor Cohn

Koch was fortunately placed in two ways. First, his nearest university was Breslau where Cohn, the well-known professor of botany was already interested in bacteria.

The 32-year old country doctor plucked up his courage and wrote to the great professor. Cohn was very doubtful that an unknown country doctor from the Polish part of Germany would have anything sensible to say. However, he invited Koch over and was won over immediately when the young doctor demonstrated his discovery (by inoculating another animal).

Within three days the news was all round the university, how Koch, working completely alone had made such a magnificent discovery. Cohn became a great supporter of Koch and helped him publish his results.

Zeiss, Ernst Abbe and the oil immersion micrscope

Second, he became friendly with Ernst Abbe, who became consultant to, and then proprietor of the Zeiss Microscope Company. The 1870s saw Abbe developing the oil immersion lens, together with the condenser that filled the lens with light. These two improvements made microscopy much more accurate and powerful.

Thus, Koch got the tools for the job a year in advance of anyone else, and his success with them made Zeiss the world leader in microscopes.

Innovative photomicrography

Koch began to experiment with photomicrography. Photography was not an easy job in those days. Plates had to be freshly made before each picture, and very long exposures were needed. Koch used the sun to illuminate his microscope (no electricity), and a clock operated 'heliograph' to follow its movement and keep it in focus. Emmy had to stay outside to warn whenever a cloud approached.

The bacteria needed staining to be seen and he adapted a method used for the photography of tapestry. 'The long exposure and unavoidable vibration of the apparatus,' he wrote, 'mean that the pictures are not satisfactory, and for the moment I must abstain from publishing them – but when improved methods allow shorter exposures I will'.

Infection studies and publication

Lister had already shown that antiseptics could prevent wound infections, but the details of the pathology were not clear.

Koch set to work studying infections in animals with the aid of his microscope and came up with the finding – hitherto unknown – that different types of bacteria could be involved. Sorting them out was still problematic, because there was no way of separating them in laboratory cultures.

However, he was able to do so in animals, and demonstrate their presence with his special microscope with the oil immersion lens and condenser. He was still alone in Wollstein and feeling increasingly isolated … 'many new things have been reported, which I in my isolated corner of Germany know nothing about' he wrote.

His little book on *Aetiology of traumatic infective diseases* came out in 1878. By 1880 there was an English translation thanks to a King's College Hospital Surgeon called Watson Cheyne (Lister's assistant). Cheyne said that no one could doubt this work provided they believed the illustrations. 'I am able to give the most satisfactory confirmatory evidence,' he wrote, because since the book had been published Koch had sent Lister some photographs, which served to prove the accuracy of his drawings.

The call from Berlin

Koch's fame was spreading, and he was becoming increasingly frustrated at being in the backwoods.

However on 7 July 1889 he received a telegram about a research post in Berlin, 'Please reply immediately on your starting date' it read. He replied at once, 'I will be at your disposal in Berlin on 10 July.' The family held a garden sale, and took almost nothing (not even the incubator) with them to Berlin.

Plate culture development

Within only a year of starting at the Imperial Health Office in Berlin, Robert had become the leader of a very talented team, which had already laid the foundations for what is still the major technology used in today's bacteriology laboratories.

He recognised its value at once and wrote: 'The plate culture is the foundation of all research on infectious disease'. In Breslau, Koch had met Joseph Schroeter, a botanist who had studied the growth of bacteria on potatoes (see Chapter 25). The chance observation of colour on old potatoes had led to the realisation that some bacteria when growing on a surface would produce coloured colonies.

Koch realised here was the answer to a problem that worried bacteriologists for some time – how to separate out different types of bacteria from a mixture when growing them in the laboratory.

Lister had indeed prepared pure cultures of bacteria in broth. What he did (with the aid of his liqueur glasses) was to dilute out his material until it only contained a single living bacterium. This would then grow as a pure clone in broth. Not a very easy technique when one may start with literally tens of millions of bacteria in a cubic centimeter of broth.

Koch took some colonies of bacteria that had developed on the surface of a boiled potato and spread them onto slices from a second one. The slices were incubated in a moist chamber, and the bacteria grew as pure cultures.

This was all very well for bacteria that grow on potatoes, but not too good for human disease producers, which do not. The latter grew well in rich meat broth, so the problem was to combine the solid surface with the food. Again, the kitchen came in handy – he developed the idea of using gelatin as a gelling agent, in small glass dishes.

This worked very well, but had the unfortunate disadvantage that gelatin liquefies at body temperature – which is of course the temperature that human disease-producing bacteria like most of all.

Fannie Hesse and the development of agar as a gelling agent

Koch's fame was by now attracting scientists eager to work with him in Berlin. For six months in the winter of 1881, Walther Hesse worked in Koch's laboratory. His job was to study germs in the air, but most of this was done at home later, where, like Koch he was blessed with a most helpful wife – Fannie (see Figure 4), who acted as the artist for his papers, and also as his technician.

The pair of them became very frustrated in the following summer, when Koch's gelatin culture medium melted. Fannie always used agar (from Japanese seaweed) in her fruit jellies, having been taught to do so by her mother, who got the idea from Dutch friends recently returned from Indonesia. She suggested trying it as the gelling agent for the broth.

It was a great success, and so Hesse wrote and told Koch about it. The latter quickly turned over to using agar, although no paper

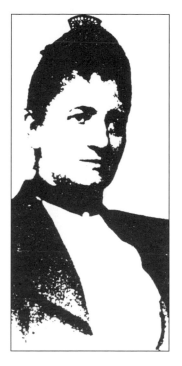

Figure 4   Fannie Hesse, the originator of agar gelling agents

on the topic was ever published, and not until years later did Fannie receive proper recognition.

Steam sterilisation and disinfection

The role of the Imperial Health Office was as a national Public Health Laboratory, so that the generation of methods for sterilisation and disinfection were an important part of their work.

On a more down to earth basis – it was no good having all these wonderful techniques for growing bacteria if they were spoilt by use of infected

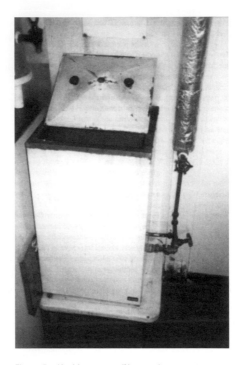

Figure 5   Koch's steamer (Newsom)

culture medium; and also the cultures need safe disposal. So the next thing was the study of heat as a sterilising agent, and the development of Koch's steamer (see Figure 5).

By now Koch had matured into the head of a very successful state department. He was no longer the enthusiastic amateur, but the self-confident professional – able to say that Pasteur's work was 'rubbish' with aplomb. Although he had achieved much, he was only at the start of things.

Further reading
Brock TP. (1998) *Robert Koch. A life in medicine and bacteriology.* Madison, Science Tech Publishers.

Chapter 7

Robert Koch, father of medical microbiology part 2: 1890–1910

Introduction

In the last chapter we saw how Robert Koch spurned the chance of fame and fortune in the US to become a doctor in an obscure country town in order to marry and support Emmy, his original girlfriend.

His desire to travel remained dormant, but encouraged by Emmy, he used his spare time to undertake research on infections – often in the most primitive conditions. He gained recognition locally through the university, and then seized the opportunity to move to Berlin when offered the leadership of the National Hygiene team – moving there with three days' notice after holding a 'garden sale' of his possessions.

Sterilisation and disinfection

Koch now had the technology to grow bacteria and the knowledge that bacterial spores were more resistant to killing than bacterial cells. One of his first jobs was to assess disinfection and sterilising processes. 'Experience,' he wrote, 'has shown the uselessness of seeking for universal disinfectants'. Too true! Lister's carbolic acid proved to be unsatisfactory for killing bacteria, although it did prevent their multiplication (on hearing this, Lister changed his policy).

Koch used a steam-heated oven to study hot-air sterilisation (no electricity), and observed that the temperature varied at different spots within the oven (modern ovens have fans to maintain an even mix of air, thereby producing a uniform temperature distribution).

Koch noted that exposure to 137°C for one hour did not kill his spores, but did damage materials such as silk, cotton, gauze and buckskin. He concluded that 140°C for three hours was required for sterilisation. Steam under pressure in primitive autoclaves had been used by the food canning industry for many years and observation showed that it worked.

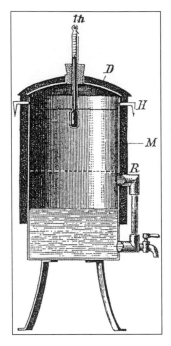

Figure 1   The plant used by Koch to kill bacteria in early experiments. This used air heated by steam, and the thermometer (th) measured the temperatures achieved. (Thomas Brock)

Koch and his colleagues used test strips containing anthrax spores, or 'earth bacteria' (the predecessor of *Bacillus stearothermophilus* spore strips) to try out different autoclave cycles. The plant they used is shown in Figure 1. They measured temperature, but not pressure, and concluded that exposure to 120°C for 20 minutes was an adequate sterilisation process.

So far so good – however, they then turned their attention to 'flowing steam' using the steamer shown in Figure 2. Here they 'went off the rails', concluding: 'In every respect exposure to flowing steam at 100°C is more certain, simpler, more rapid and economical and involves less damage to the load'. Nonetheless, their steam heating work put the whole study of sterilising processes on a firm basis.

Discovering the cause of tuberculosis

The year 1882 is almost as important for infectious disease studies as 1066 is in English history. This was the year Koch discovered the tubercle bacillus and proved it was the cause of tuberculosis.

At this time tuberculosis was a dread disease – 'galloping consumption' was the fate of many, including the young, medically-trained poet Keats, who wrote: 'That drop of blood [in his spit] is my death warrant, I must die.' He did so a year later at the age of 25. At that time around one in seven of the London population died from the disease.

Koch was able to stain the bacteria, grow them in pure culture and reproduce the disease by injecting them into animals. In so doing he developed 'Koch's postulates' – proof that a particular infection had a specific microbial cause. Even today, these are regarded as the gold standard for determining the causes of infections.

He stained the bacteria with a mixture of methylene blue and caustic potash, and grew them on inspissated beef serum. He set up 43 cultures and infected 79 guinea pigs, 35 rabbits and four cats with human material, then more animals from the cultures.

All this was achieved in just eight months, which is remarkable, especially as cultures of the tubercle bacteria take up to six weeks to grow.

Koch announces his results

In August 1882 Koch felt sure enough of his results to give a talk explaining his findings. However, the doyen of German pathology – the great Virchow – did not hold with this new-fangled bacteriology, and so Koch arranged to lecture to the members of the Berlin Physiological Society, rather than medical researchers.

He gave a very carefully thought-out talk, and in those pre-audiovisual aid days took along his actual microscope slides and cultures (preserved in alcohol) for the audience to see. When he finished there was a stunned silence: the audience was simply overwhelmed by what they had heard. Koch had discovered the cause of a widespread and deadly disease and put its diagnosis on a scientific footing.

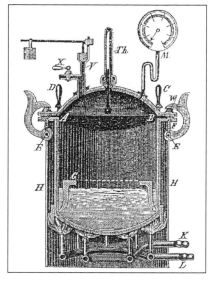

Figure 2   A cross-section of a 'flowing steam' steamer. More sophisticated than the plant of Figure 1, this equipment features a manometer for pressure measurements (M) and a weight-controlled safety valve (V) (Thomas Brock)

International recognition

Koch had expected some opposition, but there was none. Instead, the results spread quickly around the world. Within three weeks of the publication of his paper, one of his English champions had written a summary for *The Times,* which appeared a few weeks later in *The New York Times.* The latter was disturbed at the slow spread of the message: 'It is safe to say that the little pamphlet which was left to find its way through the slow mails to an English scientist outweighs in importance and interest all the dispatches which have since been flashed around the world. Items such as the progress or receding of sundry royal gouts are given to the wings of lightning, but a lumbering mail coach is swift enough for news of one of the great scientific discoveries of the age.'

People around the world were quick to look for the tubercle bacteria – a doctor in the Brompton Hospital in London (still a centre for chest disease) found a good correlation between bacilli in the sputum and clinical disease. Furthermore, he suspended glycerine-coated slides in the flues of the hospital, thereby exposing them to air at a velocity of 300–400 feet per minute from wards containing infected patients. He wished to obtain 'a concentration of the exhalations', and must have been encouraged when tests on the slides showed 'abundant bacilli'.

Promotion and entry to the German establishment

Overnight Koch became internationally-known and respected. Kaiser Wilhelm appointed him as an 'Imperial Privy Councillor', which meant an increase in salary, and entry to the establishment.

Fame resulted in a new and larger laboratory, and he no longer needed Emmy to help with his photography. He was sent abroad on an official commission to Egypt and India to look into the cause of cholera (of which more later). He became Professor of Hygiene, dividing his time between teaching, serving on commissions and working at his office desk.

The next step – from cause to control of tuberculosis

Discovery of the causative microbe was only a step towards the control of tuberculosis, and in 1889 he disappeared into the laboratory, working late and alone, with only a pile of dead guinea pigs to provide clues. Then, in 1890 out came the message: 'I have found a substance which can prevent growth of tubercle bacilli.' Koch said this at an international conference – probably before he was really ready to give full details because of political pressure.

In fact he claimed very little and had only worked on guinea pigs, but such was his fame that the world was up in arms as people flocked to Berlin for the cure. Lister took his niece for treatment and returned saying that the results were 'astounding'.

Conan Doyle visited Berlin and wrote: 'It is at present much easier to see the bacillus of Koch, than to catch the most fleeting glimpse of its illustrious discoverer' (see Figure 3). Emperor Wilhelm gave him the 'Grand Cross of the Golden Eagle' – a unique honour for a scientist.

Koch kept the details of his 'chemical' secret. Actually, it was an extract of heated tubercle bacilli. In some cases it did help to boost an individual's natural defence to tuberculosis, but in others it turned out to

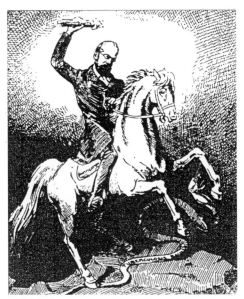

Figure 3   Koch's fame and prestige as the 'conqueror of tuberculosis' resulted in honours and even heroic cartoons (Thomas Brock)

exacerbate the illness, and it gradually became clear that it was useless for treatment. However, we still use his 'tuberculin' for diagnosis of tuberculosis.

Later, Koch made a dogmatic statement that human tuberculosis was a quite separate disease to that in the cow (shades of BSE). Unfortunately, many more people caught tuberculosis from milk until this was discredited, and milk pasteurisation began.

The foundations of a steady decline in tuberculosis – but not elimination

Koch had laid down the foundations for diagnosis and so control of tuberculosis. The death rate in Europe steadily decreased as the standard of living improved, although the infection remained quite common.

Roughly half of those my age caught tuberculosis as children (including me), but most had no severe illness. In the 1940s antibiotics and the BCG vaccine were introduced, and the incidence of the disease continued to decline. The hope was that like smallpox, tuberculosis might disappear altogether.

Sadly, though, the reverse is true today – in 1992 there were over eight million cases in the world, with an estimated 2.7 million deaths, making tuberculosis once again a 'Captain of the Men of Death'. This is mainly due to the effect of AIDS, which reduces the body's defences to infection, and occurs particularly in Africa and south-east Asia.

AIDS patients can die of the 'galloping consumption' and may be highly infectious for others.

Koch – the international researcher

In 1883, aged 41, Koch finally fulfilled his desire to travel – and at the government's expense! – when he was sent with a team to Egypt following a cholera outbreak. The Germans (and the French) badly needed to understand cholera and to prevent its spread in Europe.

Once again he acted with amazing speed. The complete equipment for a bacteriological laboratory was assembled within a week. However, on arrival in Egypt the epidemic was on the wane, but not before a member of a French team died from cholera, emphasising that this was certainly no holiday excursion.

The Germans travelled on to India, where within days of landing in Calcutta, they had obtained pure cultures of the cholera vibrio. En route Koch wrote to Emmy, saying he had also written to their 15-year-old daughter Trudy: 'To whom I have sent some stamps, flowers and a mosquito, the last so she can learn a little about the dark side of the orient'! Once again the cause of a disease – cholera – was worked out in a very short time and Koch returned in triumph to receive yet another medal from the Emperor.

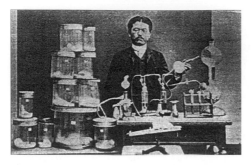

Figure 4   Researchers from all over the world such as
Shibasaburo Kitasato (above) and Lady Bruce (Chapter 19)
came to learn from Robert Koch (Thomas Brock)

By now Koch's reputation was at a peak, and many came to be taught at his new institute. For example, Shibasaburo Kitasato travelled from Japan (see Figure 4). He had already grown the tetanus bacteria, and later returned to set up a laboratory in Tokyo, where some early work on plague was done.

At home things were less settled, in the 1890s Koch became infatuated with Hedwig, one of his students, and finally Emmy left him, and returned to his family house (which he now owned). Koch married Hedwig, who accompanied him throughout his later travels. The British Colonial Office invited him to South Africa, and Figure 5 shows him in his laboratory in Kimberley working on Rinderpest, a serious cattle disease. From there he travelled to Bombay to investigate an epidemic of plague for the German Government. Then off again to New Guinea to look into malaria – all this in the 1890s, when travel was slow and facilities limited.

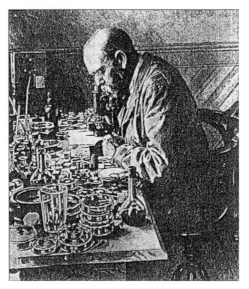

Figure 5   Koch working on Rinderpest in Kimberley,
South Africa (Wellcome Images)

Nobel prize for medicine

Koch retired in 1904, but made the trip to Stockholm in the following year to receive the Nobel prize for medicine (see Figures 6a and 6b). Even then he went back to Africa, and a final trip to the US and the Kitasato Institute in Tokyo. Not surprisingly, the degree of success had made him very self-confident to the point of arrogance, and unfortunately this backfired in the end.

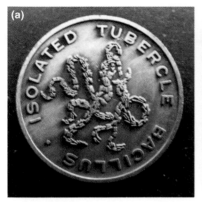
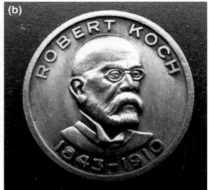

Figure 6   A Robert Koch coin from the USA (Newsom)

On his last trip to the US, a closed meeting was held at which an international group discussed whether tuberculosis could spread from the cow to the human. One of the delegates said afterwards: 'Dr Koch isolated the tubercle bacillus, today science has isolated Dr Koch.'

He returned to Berlin and commenced some further work on tuberculosis, but died soon afterwards, aged 67. A Royal Commission was set up in the UK to study the problem of bovine tuberculosis. One of the 'trusty and well beloved men' it contained was German Sims Woodhead, Professor of Pathology at Cambridge who became one of Papworth's founders. They did indeed prove that cows' milk could transmit tuberculosis to humans.

Robert Koch – founder of medical microbiology

What a life! Koch rightly deserves the title 'Founder of Medical Microbiology'. The Koch Institute in Berlin still produces excellent work on sterilisers and sterilisation, and his original labs are now a museum. It is a name that deserves to live on.

Further reading

Brock TP. (1998) *Robert Koch. A life in medicine and bacteriology.* Madison, Science Tech Publishers.

Chapter 8
Tools of the trade: the optical microscope

Introduction

In this article, rather than concentrating on an individual, I am going to look at the history of one of infection control's 'tools of the trade' – the optical microscope. The science of microscopy was one of the foundations of microbiology. For example, Lister, who was the first to grow pure cultures of bacteria (in liquid in 1877) was given a beautiful microscope by his father in 1847 (see Figure 1), and his first published works were microscopical studies. Similarly, Robert Koch, who first isolated pure cultures of bacteria on solid media (in 1881) developed a relationship with Ernst Abbe, the then owner of Carl Zeiss microscopes, and so both pioneers had access to the latest microscope technology.

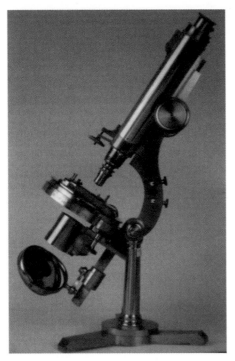

Figure 1   Joseph Lister's microscope (Royal College of Surgeons, London)

Microscopy optics

First, some simple optics: two fundamental parameters in optical microscopy are magnification (which determines the size of the image) and resolution (which is the ability to distinguish two points as separate). The physics of the eye is central to this. Objects obviously look larger the nearer they are, but for normal people about 25cm is the closest that the eye's lens can near-focus. For resolution, items have to make an angle of less than one minute of arc on the retina to be seen as separate. Resolution is in fact more important than magnification – as the latter may only produce a blur, albeit a large one. An important concept is the difference between a 'simple microscope' – or magnifying glass, which produces a virtual image (see Figure 2), and what we now call a microscope, which is in fact a 'compound microscope'. The objective lens produces a real inverted image that is then magnified into a larger virtual image by the eyepiece lens (see Figure 3). (A real image is one that can be projected onto a surface, such as a screen or photographic film).

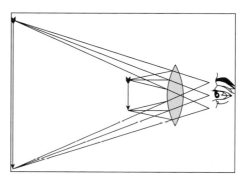

Early microscope history

The earliest origins of microscopy (from the Greek for 'small' and 'to view') are obscure. The Romans had glasses, and some ancient artefacts contain writing

Figure 2   Optical pathway for a simple microscope: the eye sees a virtual image of the arrow (Hogg, 1886)

or engraving so small that they must have required a magnifying glass to both inscribe and read. One Roman wrote: 'however small and obscure writing may be, it appears larger and clearer when viewed through a globule of glass filled with water.'

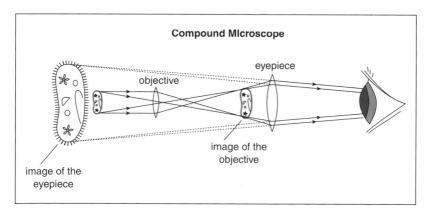

Figure 3   Optical pathway for a compound microscope (Wikipremed)

The next advances in microscopy took place in the 17th century. Credit for development should be split between Italian researchers – following Galileo and his telescope, and Dutch scientists. Galileo certainly used his telescope to look at insects – 'with this tube I have seen flies which look as big as lambs', he said. However, from our viewpoint the simple microscope was the starting point. Important contributions came from the Jesuit priest Athenasius Kircher (1602–1688). He used a 'flea glass', in which the object under study (rotting meat, soil) was stuck on a glass plate on the end of a tube. At the other end of the tube was a lens, and the whole could be pointed at a candle. Bacteria were not visible with this apparatus, because to get a high enough magnification would have required an almost spherical lens and the eye could not get close enough to such a lens to see a clear image. Nonetheless, Kircher's studies on human plague victims led him to suggest that there were corpuscles 'living or non-living ... that could allow spread of the disease by finger contact or through the air'. This is possibly the first mention of iatrogenic disease (Ayliffe & English, 2003).

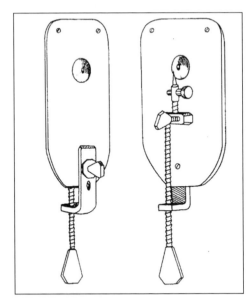

Figure 4   Leeuwenhoek's microscope (front and back views). Objects for examination were placed on the needle tip

Leeuwenhoek

Antoni van Leeuwenhoek is credited with setting the groundwork for the study of bacteria using simple microscopes, incorporating lenses he made himself by grinding glass. The lens was held in a metal plate and the object to be studied was held in front of it on a movable pinhead (see Figure 4). Leeuwenhoek. who lived in Delft, Holland from 1632 to 1723, was originally a draper. Using his microscopes he described 'small animalcules, and little eels'. He noted rods, and cocci in saliva and rainwater and protozoa. Although he did not relate these to disease, he noted that pepper and wine vinegar killed them. He was honoured by being made a Fellow of The Royal Society in London, to which he bequeathed 26 of the 500 or so instruments he had made. Recent analysis shows that the lenses approached the highest possible degree of accuracy and the best could resolve items 1 to 3.5 microns apart (the *streptococcus* has a diameter of 2 microns).

Leeuwenhoek's microscopes probably represent the fullest development of the simple microscope possible at the time. However, there was no provision for light to illuminate the object being studied – he probably pointed it at the window (or a candle), and the whole was handheld and focused by a coarse screw thread. Later developments included a mirror to concentrate light on the object, a stand, and a fine screw-thread focusing system.

Compound microscope

The compound microscope, a much more complex instrument, was first fully developed in England by Robert Hooke, whose book *Micrographia* published in 1665 did much to stimulate interest in the minute world around us. Hooke designed a compound microscope with a good stand, simple focusing and a complex stage to allow accurate placing and movement of the object, which nonetheless had to be lit from above. Fortunately, he was good at drawing and his studies of the point of a needle, the surface of a nettle leaf, and a flea, are fascinating. Later he demonstrated cells in plants, but did not understand their significance. Hooke worked in Oxford, but became Secretary of the Royal Society, and was ordered by them 'to bring at least one microscopical observation to every meeting'. However, he did not study micro-organisms.

In fact, bacteria would have been hard for Hooke to see for two reasons connected with the properties of lenses, namely spherical aberration and chromatic aberration. To get the best resolution, the objective lens needs to be nearly spherical, but then the rays of light passing through the outer rim are focussed to a different spot than those passing through its centre, so creating a blurred image. In Hooke's day the only answer was to block out the peripheral rays passing through the edge of the lens using a 'stop', thus reducing the efficiency of the lens. Chromatic aberration refers to the fact that different colours of the spectrum are focussed at different points. The focal point for blue light is nearer the lens than that for red, thus an image might have coloured haloes.

Most microscopists made their own lenses by grinding glass to the correct shape, which was a very exacting process. In the 1670s powdered flint was used in glass making to produce flint glass, which was easier to work. However the real advance came in 1676 when George Ravenscroft discovered that by adding lead oxide to the glass mixture it became much clearer and much easier to work.

Ravencroft's 'Christaline Glass resembling Rock Christall' was far superior to previous recipes. It was softer and easier to decorate, but most importantly it had a higher refractive index, giving it more brilliance and beauty and making it invaluable to the optical industry for the production of optical lenses for astronomical telescopes and of course microscopes. Its different refractive index (how much it bends light) fostered the idea of compound lenses – gluing two different lenses together to reduce aberrations further.

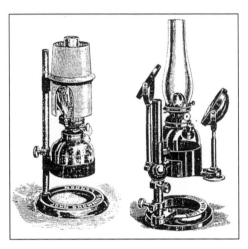

Figure 5   Early microscope lamps (Davis Practical Microscopy, 1889)

Lister and achromatic lenses

A major step in the development of microscopes for microbiology came from Lister's father – Joseph Jackson Lister. He was a wine merchant, but became fascinated by optics when as a boy he noticed that looking through air bubbles in window panes improved his vision. From 1824 to 1837 he experimented with lens combinations to produce achromatic lenses – i.e. ones with no chromatic aberration. In 1833 he was elected to the Royal Society for his achievements – unusual for a wine merchant, but illustrative of the contributions of Victorian 'amateur scientists'. His gift to his son Joseph was a 'state-of-the-art' microscope (see Figure 1), and the motivation and training to put it to good use. As well as the new lenses, it had a stage on which the object under study was placed, and below the stage was a means of transillumination. This consisted of a mirror to catch light from a window or a lamp (see Figure 5), and a condenser – a simple lens to concentrate the light on the object. If the ambient light conditions were good enough then this lens could be omitted; in which case the other side of the mirror was a convex shape, used to focus the light on the object. This of course would not work if the condenser was in place.

Joseph Lister (see Chapter 3) put the microscope to good use. His first research, done while still a medical student on 'contractility of the iris', and muscle in the skin (goose pimples) was published in 1853 in the *Royal Microscopical Society Journal*.

In the early 1870s he reported on the structure of yeasts and bacteria, grown in his 'glass garden' (see Figure 6). His papers were illustrated by fine drawings (see Figure 7), and supported his work on the 'germ theory of putrefaction'. He also described *Penicillium glaucum.* which he noted produced a musty smell, but he did not associate it with antimicrobial activity, thus missing the chance of finding penicillin.

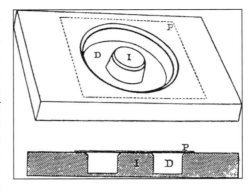

Figure 6   Lister's 'glass garden'. The trough was filled with growth medium and covered with a glass square

Koch

Robert Koch had saved to buy the best microscope he could while still an obscure GP. In 1873 he studied blood from a sheep that had died of anthrax, and noted the presence of spores. This work set him on the road to success, and spurred him on – his family and indeed everything else came second to his research. His wife wrote: 'Through careful saving of money a better microscope was obtained.' Koch's Uncle Edward had encouraged an interest in photography during his youth, and now he wanted to take photographs of his microscopic preparations, which he thought would be more accurate than drawings. He obtained the best

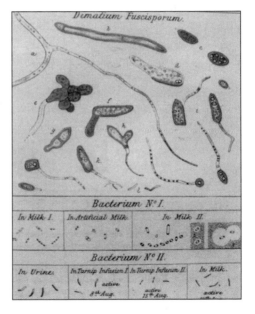

Figure 7   Lister's drawings of microbes (1873)

equipment available, but even then could not get more than a 300x magnification (Leeuwenhoek's best lens provided 275x magnification). Photography involved making your own fresh plates (the predecessors of film) and very long exposures. Koch even made a clock operated mirror outside his window to ensure a continuous supply of sunlight.

Fortunately for Koch, another German – Ernst Abbe (1840 to 1905) had left his job as lecturer at Jena University to become a consultant to (and later proprietor of) the Carl Zeiss Microscope Company. The study of bacteria required more powerful microscopes, and Abbe found that by using oil between the lens and the microscope slide – light could be concentrated, and higher power lenses could be used giving magnifications of up to 1000 times. Later he designed a much better condenser system to provide his high power lens with more light. In 1878 Koch visited Abbe and obtained one of the first oil-immersion lenses ever made, and this helped considerably in his work. Abbe wrote: 'as a proof of excellence of definition… are the favourable results which Dr Koch of Wollstein obtained when examining bacteria.' Later he developed lenses made of fluorite instead of glass. These were easier and cheaper to make, and he called them apochromatic (in contrast to achromatic).

Microscopy and dyes

Bacteria are fairly colourless and not readily seen, and in the presence of opaque matter such as blood or body tissues they may be invisible. However, Koch learnt that aniline dyes (such as methyl violet) could be used to stain most bacteria, and so make them easier to pick out. The right concentration of dye was needed, followed by a good rinse process to remove the excess. This work helped him with his most important discovery, that of the tubercle bacillus in 1882.

Today, we rarely use Koch's name in our work, although he spent a lifetime laying its foundations. Paradoxically, the name of Hans Christian Gram (1853 to 1938) is used daily in laboratories throughout the world. Gram was a Danish histologist who spent a few months in the public mortuary in Berlin with Dr Friedlander, trying to stain tissue sections from the lungs of those who had died of pneumonia to demonstrate cocci. He too used aniline dies, but then fixed these with iodine, decolourised with absolute alcohol, and suggested a counterstain of 'Bismark brown' for the tissue. In his original paper (Gram, 1884) he noted that the cocci stained blue, but that typhoid bacilli were easily decolourised (even after being immersed in stain for 24 hours). The paper had an 'editor's note' – that the Gram method was one of the best he had tried. Having succeeded in his project of differentiating the cocci from lung tissue, Gram returned to Denmark and never again dabbled in bacteriology.

Some bacteria do not hold any stain at all – especially the spirochaetes that cause syphilis. One way to visualise these is by use of 'dark field' microscopy. A special condenser is used to provide oblique rays (see Figure 8). When an object (such as a spirochaete) is hit by these rays they are directed upwards through the microscope. One of my earliest jobs (SHO in pathology) was collection of samples from the venereal disease clinic to examine by dark-field microscopy.

In those far-off days syphilis was quite rare (even in London) and if I did find the spirochaetes I had the privilege of buying the laboratory staff a walnut layer cake for tea to celebrate!

Modern microscopes

So we come to the present day – we still use the oil-immersion lens, but now the microscopes have binocular eyepieces, and are more comfortable to use. For further reading: *The Microscope – Past and Present* (Bradbury 1968), is recommended. Once again I have skimmed over the topic – no mention of phase-contrast, fluorescence or electron microscopy – all used in today's laboratories.

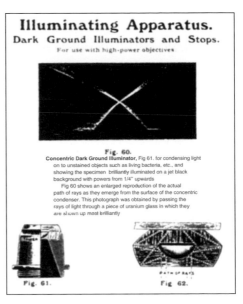

Figure 8 Example of a dark field condenser (advertisement taken from the catalogue of (C. Baker, Microscopes)

Acknowledgement

I am grateful to the Royal College of Surgeons, London for the photograph of Lister's Microscope.

Further reading

Ayliffe GAJ. English MP. (2003) *Hospital Infection, from Miasmas to MRSA.* Cambridge University Press: Cambridge.

Bradbury S. (1968) *The Microscope. Post and Present.* Pergamon Press: Oxford.

Brock TD. (1988) *Robert Koch. A life in Medicine and Bacteriology.* Science Tech Publishers: Madison.

Gram C. (1884) *Ueber die isolirte Farbung der Schizomyceten in Schnitt-und Trockenparapten. Fortschritte der Medicin.* **2**: 185–9. (The differential staining of Schizomycetes in tissue sections and dried preparations: translated by the American Society for Microbiology and available on the Internet under 'Christian Gram').

Lister J. (1909) *The collected works of Joseph Baron Lister.* Clarendon Press: Oxford, (reprinted in the *Classics of Medicine Library.* Birmingham: Alabama.).

Chapter 9
Smallpox: an infection controlled

Introduction

Back in my student days again (I am in my dotage!), I remember the Professor saying: 'you will remember this name all your life even though it is quite irrelevant to exams or modern medicine – Lady Mary Wortley Montagu.' I certainly did. Now I have had time to read about her, I realise what an amazing person she must have been.

However, first things first. A less well-known name is Ali Maow Maalin, the Somali cook who in 1977 became the world's last naturally acquired case of smallpox.

Smallpox epidemics

Smallpox is unique in having been eradicated from the world. In the middle ages it was the cause of one of the major epidemics. Ten thousand cases were recorded in the London boroughs between 1901 and 1904. Some 75% of these people had been vaccinated (10% died) and 25% were unvaccinated (32% died). Even in 1923 there were 110,000 cases in the US.

The disease produced terrible 'pocks' (see Figure 1), and even if you survived you would be scarred for life. However, two points stood out: the infection was restricted to humans and if you recovered you were then immune. The last point was so well known that an advertisement for a servant would typically read something like: 'Wanted: a man between 20 and 30 years as footman for a great family. He must be Church of England, and have had the smallpox in a natural way.'

The development of vaccination

The Chinese used intentional infection for protection of children, and 'sowed the pox' using powdered scabs as snuff. This must have been very risky, as the dose was uncontrolled and the full-blown illness might occur.

Not until Edward Jenner realised that milkmaids infected with cowpox were immune to smallpox and popularised 'vaccination' (vacca means cow) did a really safe way to prevent the disease gain general acceptance. In 1996, the 200th anniversary of the vaccination of James Phipps by Jenner was marked by many celebrations (see Chapter 10).

Jenner was a Gloucestershire country doctor and his house at Berkeley has become the 'Jenner Museum', which is well worth a visit. Although he rightly gets the credit for the eradication of smallpox. I want to focus on two of his predecessors who played a significant part in the story. Lady Mary Wortley Montagu and Benjamin Jesty.

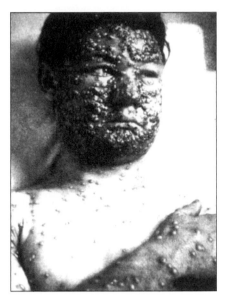

Figure 1   Smallpox produced terrible 'pocks' on victims' skin

Lady Mary Wortley Montagu

Lady Mary Wortley Montagu was a very talented and outspoken lady who married Edward Wortley Montagu, the MP for Huntingdon. She did this despite the wishes of her father Lord Dorchester (a rich and powerful man). As he refused permission, she eloped (her idea) with Edward, having given him due warning: 'Reflect now for the last time in what manner you must take me. I shall come to you with only a nightgown and petticoat, and that is all you will get with me.' This was stirring stuff for the year 1712.

Not long after, she was left in Hinchingbrooke House – the hospital is now in its grounds – with her 'in-laws', while her husband was in London and she was expecting their first child. She was miserable. She wrote, 'I opened a closet where I hoped to find many books, but to my great disappointment there were only some pieces of law and folios of mathematics, my Lord Hinchingbrook having disposed of the rest. I walked yesterday on the terrace for two hours.'

A year later her brother died of smallpox, and she herself had an attack, which somewhat dimmed her beauty. These happenings almost certainly set the stage for the future. In 1716 she accompanied her husband, who had been appointed as ambassador, to Turkey. Her letters recorded the manners and customs of Turkish ladies, and she took to wearing Turkish dress (as we saw in the Introduction, page 4).

However, her most relevant experience was to become acquainted with the widely used practice of inoculation. To a friend she wrote: 'Apropos of distempers, I am going to tell you a thing that I am sure will make you wish you were here. People send to one another to know if any of their family has a mind to have the smallpox; they make parties attended by an old woman with a nut-shell of the matter of the best form of smallpox, who asks what veins you wish opened.'

Within the year, she was so convinced of its value that she had her son Edward inoculated and, on her return to London, persuaded her physician Dr Maitland to set up as an 'inoculator'. This 'heathen rite' drew antipathetic sermons, together with abuse from the medical faculty.

However, Lady Mary persisted and obtained powerful support from Dr Richard Mead, whose book on the topic later ran into seven editions (in Latin). In 1721 she obtained permission for a 'clinical trial' on seven condemned criminals. Thereafter inoculation went from strength to strength. When two members of the royal family underwent the operation successfully, it became the fashion.

Lady Mary and her family were truly amazing. In 1739, after 27 years of married life, she took off to Italy, where she remained until 1760. Then her husband's death (aged 83) made her think of home and she made the arduous journey back, but did not live more than a year longer.

Her son Edward, despite his father's meanness (the latter died a millionaire – old miser himself), was the prototype of the 'Rake's Progress'. He married at least three times, firstly a dairymaid, then twice bigamously. Like his father he became the MP for Huntingdon, which did not stop him being imprisoned in Paris for gambling debts, and he ended back in Turkey living an idle life. 'I have never committed a small folly,' he boasted. His parents still corresponded, and when his father was considering writing yet another letter to him (at the time living with a 'tutor' in Holland) to stop his allowance, he sent a draft of the letter to Lady Mary in Italy for her comments before sending it on to Holland – and all this in the 1750s (long before the invention of email!).

Lady Mary clearly had great determination and powers of observation, together with a lively mind and ability to document her feelings. There is a recent Penguin book entitled *The selected letters of Lady Mary Wortley Montagu.* She was a friend of princes and poets, and expressed ideas of education and rights for women that were centuries before her time.

If she could walk today on the terrace at Hinchingbrooke she would see no graves or scarred faces, and could take a significant part of the credit for this.

Benjamin Jesty

Benjamin Jesty (see Figure 2) was a Dorset farmer who lived in Yetminster, then in Worth Matravers. In 1774, some 20 years before Jenner's experiment, he was

living on the farm at Yetminster with his wife
and children while a smallpox epidemic was
raging around.

Also on the farm were the two milkmaids
Mary and Ann who, like others of their profession, were traditionally called 'fair of face'
because of having had cowpox. This was not
a serious illness, but they were known to be
immune to smallpox. Indeed, both had
nursed relatives through attacks of smallpox
without catching it.

Benjamin had also had cowpox, but was
very worried about his wife and children.
He knew that there was an outbreak of
cowpox on the next farm, so persuaded his
wife to take the children across. He used a
stocking needle to scratch material from a
'mature' pock onto his wife's arm just

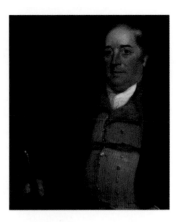

Figure 2   Benjamin Jesty (Wellcome
Images)

below the elbow, then on to those of his two little boys. Elizabeth became
very ill indeed, her arm was inflamed and she was feverish. Her doctor said:
'You have done a bold thing Mr Jesty, but I will get you through if I can' (my
guess is the doctor was referring to the charge of murder if things had gone
badly).

Fortunately Elizabeth survived, but Benjamin was regarded as an inhuman
brute by the neighbours – so much so that the family moved off to the delightful village of Worth Matravers (not far from Swanage) shortly afterwards. His
vaccination obviously worked however, because the churchyard has both his
grave and that of Elizabeth, which show that she lived to the age of 84 (Benjamin
had lived to be 79).

Rewards and recognition

Perhaps we would not have known about Benjamin but for the arrival in 1801 of
a new vicar called Dr Bell in Swanage. Dr Bell was very keen on vaccination and
was disappointed that it was not much in use locally. During his enquiries he
met with Benjamin and heard about his feat.

Possibly the fact that Jenner had been awarded £10,000 may have stimulated
Benjamin to reveal what he had previously kept quiet about, or perhaps it was
pride in doing something that was now respectable. Anyway he was duly invited
to the 'Vaccine pock' Institute in London, and presented with a pair of gold-
mounted lancets and a testimonial.

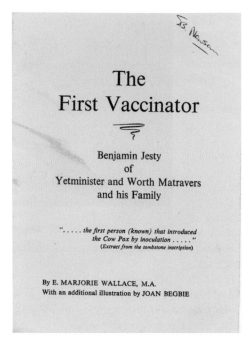

The First Vaccinator

Benjamin Jesty
of
Yetminister and Worth Matravers
and his Family

".....the first person (known) that introduced
the Cow Pox by inoculation ....."
(Extract from the tombstone inscription)

By E. MARJORIE WALLACE, M.A.
With an additional illustration by JOAN BEGBIE

Figure 3   The stroy of Benjamin Jesty (available in the chruch at Worth Matravers)

So despite Jenner's annoyance, Benjamin was recognised, and I think he was quite satisfied, because his aim all along had been for health and happiness for his family, and in this he clearly succeeded.

Conclusion

It is of course a large jump from the Jesty family to the whole world. The efforts of the World Health Organization in managing to cross all national, political and cultural frontiers in the 1970s to both ensure widespread vaccination and then monitor the last remaining cases of the disease is truly amazing.

Clearly, where a disease is strictly affecting humans' and immunisations can be used, we can look forward to the disappearance of other infections. Indeed, Luis Fermin (a Peruvian baby) was the last person in the Americas to develop paralytic poliomyelitis, and measles eradication is also well under way. A truly amazing scenario, which seemed unbelievable even 50 years ago.

Further reading

Robert Halsband. *The Life of Lady Mary Wortley Montagu.* Oxford, Clarendon Press, 1956.
Selected Letters of Lady Mary Wortley Montagu. Edited by Robert Halsband, Harmondsworth, Penguin Books, 1970.
Doris Hastie. *A toast to Lady Mary.* London, Companion Book Club, 1955. [There are many other books on Lady Mary available]
Marjorie Wallace. *The first vaccinator. Benjamin Jesty of Yetminster and Worth Matravers.* Lobster Cottage, Worth Matravers, 1981. (Available as a monograph in the Church of St Nicholas of Myra, Worth Matravers, Dorset – the church itself is well worth a visit).

Chapter 10
The life of Edward Jenner, 1749–1823

Introduction

My previous article on smallpox (Chapter 9) set the scene. Lady Mary Wortley Montague introduced 'variolation' – inoculation of material from the 'pocks' of one suffering mild smallpox into the skin. The aim was to produce a mild attack of the illness followed by immunity. This had significant mortality, but became accepted after the Queen had had two princesses inoculated in 1722, and was endorsed by the Royal College of Physicians in 1745. Variolation was performed expertly by a few doctors, who in return made big money from those who could pay. Dr Dimsdale received £10,000 (1770s money) and £500 a year for life from the Empress of Russia. In 1746 a smallpox and inoculation institute was opened for the poor on the site of what is now St Pancras station in London and variolation became more widely used.

The popular concept of Edward Jenner (see Figure 1) is of a quiet country GP. Nothing could be further from the truth. He was born into a large family in 1749. His father was vicar of Berkeley, but also a landowner rich enough to send his two eldest sons to Oxford. Both parents died before Edward was five, so his sisters brought him up. Aged eight he went to the free school in Wotton-

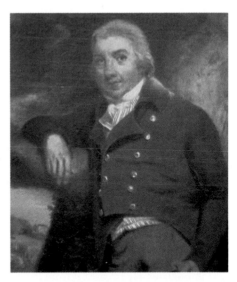

Figure 1   Edward Jenner (1749–1823) painted by William Pearce (The Jenner Museum, Berkeley)

under-Edge, where he boarded with the headmaster and during a smallpox epidemic underwent 'variolation'. This involved six weeks of purges until he was emaciated, inoculation, and then removal to 'an inoculation stables where he was haltered up with others in a terrible state of disease, although none died'. This must have made a major impression on him.

Education

Although interested in natural sciences, he decided on medicine. There was enough family money for him to become an apprentice surgeon when he was twelve years old. His apprenticeship lasted six years and he could have earned a living (provided he did not practise in London or Edinburgh where the Colleges of Surgeons ruled). However, he made an inspired move – he became a student of John Hunter, London's leading surgeon, an experimental scientist of note. By May 1772 he had obtained a certificate from Hunter stating he 'hath diligently attended four courses of my anatomical and chirurgical lectures'. He was now better educated than if he had been to Oxford or Cambridge – the only two centres allowed to train physicians. He made many contacts in London, including Joseph Banks, the botanist who had been on Captain Cooke's voyage around the world and later became President of the Royal Society. At Hunter's suggestion, Jenner helped Banks to catalogue his collection of plants. Hunter wanted Jenner to become his partner, and Banks offered him the post of botanist for Cooke's last voyage. However, he refused both as he relished the country life.

Jenner returned to Berkeley and lived in the vicarage with his brother Stephen, who was the vicar. He was easily the most qualified surgeon around, and developed a practice covering about 400 square miles including both Gloucester and Cheltenham, travelling on horseback whatever the weather. He had enough private income to enjoy his scientific pursuits, and influential friends and mentors in London. For 20 years he corresponded with Hunter – the Royal College of Surgeons has a collection of Hunter's letters, but sadly only one of Jenner's replies. Hunter's letters included advice on wide-ranging topics. 'Don't just think about it, try the experiment' or 'forget the woman, she wouldn't have been worth it'.

Scientific progress

Jenner's scientific interests were extensive. His hydrogen balloon was one of the first in England. He released it from the grounds of Berkeley Castle, and it flew to Birdlip where to this day the landing is marked by the 'Air Balloon' Inn. Hibernation was a major interest. Hunter demanded hedgehogs and sent Jenner a thermometer (with instructions) to measure their temperatures. In 1783 Jenner worked out a way to purify tartar emetic (still in the pharmacopoeia and used until recently for schistosomiasis and leishmaniasis), and later showed that angina sufferers had calcified coronary arteries. This was a difficult one, as he knew that Hunter suffered from angina, and did not wish him to be upset by these findings. He also studied the properties of human blood as a fertiliser!

More to the point was his interest in birds. He studied cuckoos' breeding habits and showed that the baby cuckoo ejected the other inhabitants from the nest. This was a major discovery, one that caused a controversy that was not settled until cine-photography became available in the 1920s. However, it earned him the coveted Fellowship of the Royal Society. He did not subscribe to the prevailing theory that birds spent the winter buried in the mud. Swallows reappeared in the spring looking much too fresh and he deduced that they must have migrated.

By 1785 Jenner was settled in Berkeley and bought (for £600) a very pleasant house near the church called Chantry Cottage, now the Jenner Museum (see Figure 2), and well worth a visit. Three years later he married Catherine Kingscote, from the neighbouring village of that name. Her family seem to have taken years to accept Edward as a suitable partner. They had a good life together, but sadly she died of tuberculosis in 1815; their eldest son, Edward, also died from tuberculosis in 1810. In 1792 he finally became 'Doctor Jenner' with a degree from St Andrews, where the practice of selling them to those who had suitable referees was still in force! As a family man Jenner needed more income and comfortable surroundings, so he obtained a house and practised in Cheltenham (even then a spa town), keeping Chantry Cottage as his permanent home.

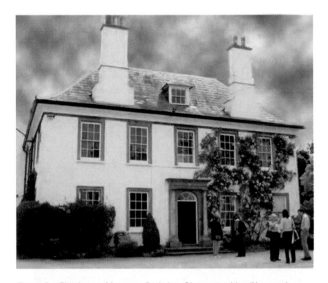

Figure 2   The Jenner Museum, Berkeley, Gloucestershire (Newsom)

Vaccination

Jenner had always been interested in cowpox and like Benjamin Jesty observed that those who had had cowpox did not get smallpox. In his first publication (*The Inquiry*, 1798) he noted that his interest went back 25 years, and indeed he had mentioned it to Hunter when he was a student. Jenner had a very powerful tool available – variolation. He did not need to wait for a smallpox epidemic to see who was immune. He could see if the variola virus would 'take' when he inoculated it. Jenner used the word virus, although at the time no one knew what it was. Virus meant 'poison'. Indeed today's germs were originally called 'filterable viruses' – as they passed through filters known to block bacteria.

In 1789 a mild eruptive fever called variously swinepox, pigpox or cowpox appeared in Gloucester. The nurse attending Jenner's young son Edward developed the disease. Jenner took material from her to inoculate Edward and two servants (thus emulating Benjamin in his desire to protect his own family). A month later he challenged all three with variola, and showed they were immune.

However his definitive experiment was the inoculation of an eight-year-old village boy called James Phipps on 14 May 1796 with material from a cowpox lesion on the finger of Sarah Nelmes – the daughter of a local farmer. She had caught cowpox from 'Blossom' (see Figure 3), whose horns are now in the Jenner museum, and hide at St George's Hospital. Figure 4 shows Jenner's drawing of Sarah's finger, and is important because it shows single lesions – a true smallpox vesicle would have contained lots of smaller bubbles. James recovered quickly and when challenged on both arms with variola in July showed no reaction, nor did he some months later, James became Jenner's most celebrated patient, and was set up in a nearby cottage. He was repeatedly challenged over the years with variola virus, which of course never caused any reaction. Jenner used this to support his thesis that the immunity was lifelong. The fallacy in this argument was that the challenge doses would have reinforced the immunity, and his insistence on the 'lifelong' became a bone of contention.

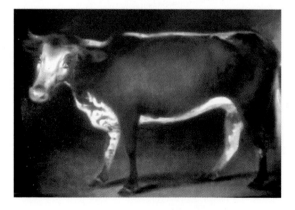

Figure 3   Blossom (The Jenner Museum, Berkeley)

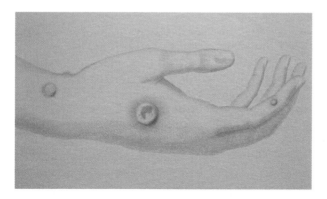

Figure 4   Sarah Elmes' arm   from *The Inquiry*

Cowpox was rare, and it was two years before another farm worker, Thomas Virgoe, caught it, seemingly from a horse. James Baker was inoculated with material from Thomas, but died before he could be challenged. Jenner was secretive about this and later ascribed the death to workhouse fever. Material from a cow with cowpox that had been milked by another farm worker who had also been infected by the horse was used to inoculate William Summers, aged five, and was transferred from him to seven others. Material from a pustule was stored for three months dried on a quill, and used with success.

The Inquiry (see Figure 5) is the basis of vaccination. It would hardly be acceptable to the Food and Drug Administration (FDA) if presented today. The evidence presented included 25 humans infected 'naturally' with cowpox, 24 of whom were resistant to smallpox, and the vaccination of nine children and an unknown number of adults and children related to one case. Only four of those vaccinated were later challenged with variola. Jenner included a discussion of two fundamental points – the signs and origin of cowpox. He differentiated the lesions (on the cow's teats) of 'true' and 'pseudo' cowpox, and he speculated that cows were infected from horses suffering from a disease of hooves called 'grease'. Horses were the equivalent of cars today, so every farm would have had lots around.

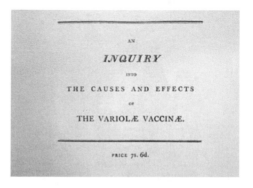

AN

INQUIRY

INTO

THE CAUSES AND EFFECTS

OF

THE VARIOLÆ VACCINÆ.

PRICE 7s. 6d.

Figure 5   *The Inquiry* – published by Jenner in 1897

Reactions to The Inquiry

Jenner had taken some dried material to London, but did not initially receive much attention. Hunter recommended he set up a practice in London where he could be assured of an income of £10,000 a year. This would not have pleased those already getting a good income from variolation, and indeed such were among the first anti-vaccinationists. (See Figure 6 for an anti-vaccination poster.) However, Jenner was not in it for the money and indeed used the 'Temple of Vaccinia', a folly in his garden at Berkeley for free vaccination clinics (see Figure 7).

Two London physicians showed immediate interest. George Pearson, a physician at St George's, quickly collected and published data to support Jenner. William Woodville was in charge of the Smallpox and Inoculation Hospital at St Pancras Here was a man whose practice was totally committed to the subject. At the end of January 1799, he heard of cowpox in the nearby farm at Grays Inn Lane. He summoned Pearson and Banks to examine the cows, and they confirmed that this was 'true' cowpox. Woodville then got to work and by May had vaccinated 600 people, some from the cow, some from a dairymaid's naturally-acquired lesion, and others by person-to-person transfer. He made a significant observation early on – he showed that the human material could be used to infect a calf.

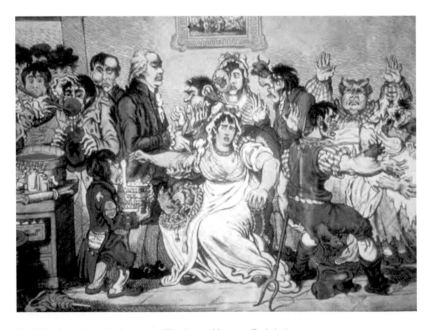

Figure 6   An anti-vaccination poster (The Jenner Museum, Berkeley)

Sadly 60% of his patients developed a generalised rash often indistinguishable from smallpox, including those originally inoculated directly from the cow, although none seem to have died. 'I used newly-ground lancets', he wrote. Although he variolated some vacinees at the same time (at the start he did not know if vaccination would work, so he continued with variolation), he took vaccine material from them before the variolation had time to work. In addition, patients were being treated for smallpox in the hospital. Thus there was a confusing set-back, and Woodville must have distrusted Jenner's work.

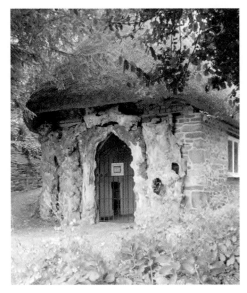

Figure 7   Temple of vaccinia (Newsom)

Controversy continued in the shape of Anne Bumpus. She was vaccinated by Woodville at three removes from a cow and developed a generalised rash. Pearson, who had developed the idea of drying vaccine on threads, sent material from her primary lesion to Jenner, who used it on some children, including his great-nephew Stephen, but did not find any generalised reactions. He was concerned, however, about inflammation around Stephen's inoculation site. Jenner thought that Woodville was using material contaminated with variola. Looked at the situation with today's knowledge, there are several other explanations. Anne could have had one of the rare generalised reactions to vaccinia still seen today, and the lancet used on Stephen could have become contaminated with *staphylococci* or even *streptococci*. Personal hygiene was not very good, and it is easy to visualise impetigo or erysipelas being transmitted with the vaccine. Even the lancet (a sort of penknife) was probably transported in the inoculator's pocket.

Spreading the news

While controversy continued for years in England, the message spread rapidly around the world. Sometimes dried matter was sent out from England, on other occasions local cows were used. Most of the time England was at war with both France and Spain. Nonetheless Woodville visited Boulogne (having had to travel via neutral Denmark) carrying some material, and soon the number of vacinees in Paris was far greater than that in London. Later Jenner wrote to Napoleon to ask for an exchange of prisoners (unheard of at the time). According to legend Napoleon said: 'Ah, Jenner, Je ne puis rien refuser a Jenner.'

Lord Elgin took vaccine from Vienna to Athens and Constantinople by having his son vaccinated, and from there it reached India, beating Jenner's plans to send material directly to India.

Perhaps the most amazing story is of the ship that sailed from Corunna in 1803 on orders from King Carlos with 'medical gentlemen', 22 healthy children and trading goods to defray expenses. One child had cowpox, and the others were inoculated sequentially. The ship stopped at the Canaries, Puerto Rico and Venezuela where the group split up, some going north to Mexico, and others across the Pacific to the Philippines and then home. Altogether at least 230,000 vaccinations were performed. Jenner commented that 'although we are at war with Spain, I have made peace and quite adore her philanthropic monarch'.

Politics

To further his interests Jenner spent a significant amount of time in London. While he was there he obtained the king's support, and eventually parliament granted him £10,000 for his expenses. He then rented a house in Hertford Street (just off Hyde Park Corner) and practised there for a while. He was only a few hundred yards from the Grosvenor Chapel, where later, Florence Nightingale (who lived three streets away) worshipped and Lady Mary Wortley Montagu was buried. Indeed he numbered Lady Mary's son-in-law among his patients. However, his income did not justify the expense and his accounts for 1799 to 1802 showed a net loss of £2,300, so he returned home.

A Royal Jennerian Society was set up as a charity with Royal patronage, and he was asked to become the president of its medical council. The aim was to provide free inoculations, but sadly it only survived a few years, being torn apart by internal politics following the doubtful behaviour of its resident inoculator.

Many other contraversies followed, but the message was spreading – parliament granted him another £20,000, and honours poured in. Business tycoons from Madras and Bombay raised £3183-1-10d. The City of London made him a freeman and gave him a gold box containing £100. Oxford University gave him an honorary doctorate of medicine. Two honours he did not get were a knighthood, and the fellowship of the Royal College of Physicians. The former was probably a reflection of royal displeasure following the demise of the Royal Jennerian Society, and the latter because he refused to fulfil the requirement for a knowledge of Latin and Greek. 'At my time of life to set about brushing up (his classical education) would be irksome to me beyond measure: I would not do it for a diadem' was his reaction.

What is vaccinia?

Jenner used several different sources for his vaccines, Blossom via Sarah, Thomas Virgoe, Ann Bumpus (from London) and others. Material was taken from cows (Benjamin Jesty) or farm workers (Woodville, Sacco in Italy). Gradually Woodville's idea of using calves to propagate the virus became generally acceptable, and in fact I was vaccinated with calf lymph.

The big riddle is: vaccinia does not cause cowpox, and is distinct from the cowpox virus in the laboratory. How did it arise? Could it have been a hybrid of variola and cowpox when both were used together on one person? The problem is made worse because variolation was banned in 1840, and smallpox virus is no longer available for study.

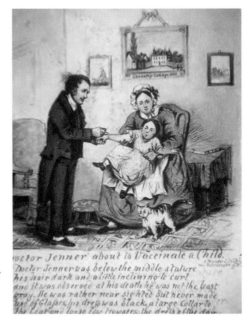

Figure 8　Cartoon of Jenner vaccinating a child, by Stephen Jenner (The Jenner Museum Berkeley)

Horsepox too has disappeared. Was horsepox modified by passage through a cow? Derek Baxby, a virologist from Liverpool wrote an excellent monograph on the topic in 1981. He concluded that there was a gradual selection from the earlier strains, so that the 20C vaccines were less toxic, and became similar. Horsepox virus he felt was a good candidate parent, but he thought we shall never know the answer.

The advent of bioterrorism and the availability of molecular biology and genetic manipulation technology have resulted in a sudden increase in research on vaccinia. A recent paper from Helsinki described a case of cowpox (Pelkonen et al. 2003) possibly acquired from a dog – so I sent an email to one of the authors, Professor Antti Vaheri – he will know the answer I thought, but his reply really just referred me back to Baxby!

Conclusion

As he grew older, Jenner spent less time in London, and gave up Cheltenham after his wife's death in 1815. He returned to the life of a country landowner in Berkeley, and continued his interest in natural history and his garden. This carried him through fits of depression about the resistance to his work. Some geologists still say that his most important work was the finding of the fossil remains of a Pleisaurus at the foot of Stinchcombe Hill in 1819 – the first in Britain. Jenner died in 1823 and was buried in the family vault at Berkeley Church – sited, probably due to his father's memory, in the key position just to the north of the altar table.

Although vaccination is probably the greatest advance towards health ever, the anti-vaccination lobby in the UK has always been very vocal. In 1896 the *British Medical Journal* devoted a whole issue to Jenner's centenary, but later noted with annoyance that in the Gloucester local elections an anti-vaccination candidate was elected. There is an excellent statue of Jenner in Kensington Gardens – sitting on a chair with the correct medical symbol, and a cow head on its side. This statue was originally in Trafalgar Square, but was moved in 1856, partly because Trafalgar Square was becoming regarded as a celebration of military triumphs, and partly in deference to the anti-vaccination lobby.

Not until the 1880s was another immunising agent introduced – by Pasteur. He was honoured by having the 'Pasteur Institute' named after him. A similar institute was later erected in London (overlooking Battersea Bridge) and for a short time was called the Jenner Institute, but again anti-vaccinationists had their say and its name became the Lister Institute. What a sad reflection on one of our greatest contributors to medicine.

Acknowledgements

I am grateful to the Jenner Museum, Berkeley for their slides and helpful comments. The museum can be contacted on: 01453 810631.

Further reading

Bazin H. (2000) *The eradication of smallpox.* Academic Press: London.

Baxby D. (1981) *Jenner's smallpox vaccine.* Heinemann: London.

Fisher RB. (1991) *Edward Jenner.* Andre Deutsch: London.

Jenner E. (1798) *An inquiry into the causes and effects of Variolae Vaccinae, a disease discovered in some of the western countries of England, particularly Gloucestershire, and known by the name of cowpox.* Printed for the author by Sampson Lowe, London. Reprinted in: *The classics of medicine library.* (1978) Birmingham, Alabama.

Pelkonen PM. Tarvainen K. Hynninen A. Kallio ERK. Henttonen H. Palva A. Vaheri A. Vapalahti O. (2003). Cowpox with severe generalized eruption. *Emerg Infect Dis* **9**: 1458–61.

Royal College of Surgeons of England. (1976) *Letters from the past from John Hunter to Edward Jenner.* Royal College of Surgeons: London.

Chapter 11

Hygiene and the Ancient Romans

Introduction

Your editors have given me a challenge; not my usual type of topic, and one that is bound to be speculative. Anyway, let me begin with mother's brooch (Figure 1) – a gift from my father when in the Royal Army Medical Corps. The snake around the staff is the symbol of Asclepius (Greek – also Aesclepius, Asklepios). He was probably a Greek physician, but became immortalised as a god – the son of Apollo. Three of his daughters were Meditirina, Hygieia (arguably the first Infection Control Practitioner) and Panacea. Temples of healing (Asclepieions) grew up around Greece, and became associated with medical schools. The snake and staff had appeared earlier – in the Book of Exodus. The Lord made Moses throw his staff on the ground, whereupon it became a serpent, reverting to a staff when Moses picked it up (by the tail). A staff surrounded by two intertwined snakes is called a caduceus and is often regarded as a medical symbol, but actually represents Hermes and so strictly should be associated with alchemy.

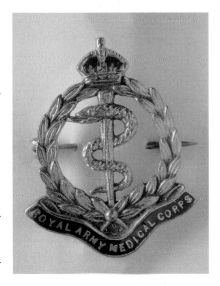

Figure 1   Aesculapius' snake and staff (Newsom)

Legend has it that during a great plague (293BC), the Romans sent to Epidaurus for Aesculapius (Roman spelling). To be sure he could not be found, but his incarnation in the form of a snake came by boat to Rome and slid off onto the boat-shaped Tiber Island (Figure 2). The plague abated and a temple to Aesculapius was built where the snake had disembarked. Sleeping in the temple, perhaps followed by a discussion of dreams with the priest, resulted in cures. Later, the Romans used to leave elderly or sickly slaves on the island to avoid

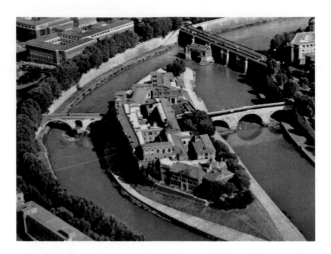

Figure 2   The Tiber island

having to care for them. Claudius enacted that abandoned slaves should be regarded as free men, and this was the start of a public hospital for the poor. This small island has always thereafter been associated with health and is happily placed upstream of the Cloaca maxima (see later). The temple has long since been covered by the Basilica in honour of San Bartomoleo, whose remains are in a covered bath, placed in front of the altar. The temple spring still feeds a well placed in the centre of the church. The principal other buildings on the island form a hospital, and here it was that the Knight Rahere swore that if he recovered from his fever (malaria) he would found another hospital – so explaining the origin of St Bartholomew's in London.

The ancient Greeks were highly developed, living in city states, excelling as philosophers and theoreticians. Hippocrates, who lived on the island of Cos, is regarded as the 'father of medicine', and assembled the first known collection (corpus) of medical literature. He is remembered in the Hippocratic oath, which begins: 'sworn by Apollo the physician, by Aesculapius, Hygieia and Panacea.' His writings on hygiene include advice on diets, and siting of 'settlements'. Before a place is colonised the soil should be examined. Marshes and swamps are to be avoided, and sunny hillsides are recommended.

The Romans revered Greek knowledge, especially in medical matters, and in 46BC Julius Caesar granted citizenship to foreign doctors, including many of Greek origin who had been brought to Rome as slaves. Antonius Musa (as mentioned in Rupert Graves' *I Claudius*) rocketed to fame in 23BC when he cured the Emperor Augustus, who thereafter made all doctors immune to taxation.

Romans were practical people, good builders and soldiers, able to manage a large empire. They knew how to make concrete (knowledge lost in the middle ages), and how to build in brick and stone. The Pantheon in Rome has an enormous concrete dome – made especially lighter at the top, which has survived since Hadrian's time (117AD). Time becomes unreal when considering the Roman era. Rome was founded in 735BC, and the era ended with the fall of Constantinople in 1453AD. However, the transfer of power from Rome to Constantinople (now Istanbul) by Constantine in 324AD marked the beginning of the decline in Rome itself. The Romans ruled Britain for 400 years following Claudius' invasion of 43AD.

Water and drainage

Aqueducts
Provision of clean water and drainage for everyone remains one of the World Health Organization's fundamental aims, one shared by the Romans. In its heyday ancient Rome had around one million inhabitants, often living in multistorey buildings. Nine aqueducts brought water from the surrounding hills, providing up to 80 gallons per head per day – similar to that in modern New York. The post of water commissioner, *Curator aquorum*, was a highly prestigious government office. Water was piped to up to 800 public baths, to fountains (used by the poor), and to the villas of the rich, who paid water rates. Aqueducts were built throughout the empire (see Figure 3). When a city could afford it, they would employ a surveyor (usually from the nearest army camp). The surveyor marked the watercourse using a dioptra, an instrument supplied with levelling sticks and plumb lines. The

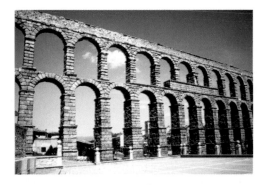

Figure 3   The aqueduct at Segovia (Mary Ann Sullivan: see www.bluffton.edu)

engineers knew that water finds its own level, so were able to build channels down steep slopes, and cross valleys. They also used syphons to good effect.

Considerable care was taken to find an unpolluted source such as a spring. Whatever the source, when the water arrived at its destination it was held in settling tanks, which by chance would have eradicated many potentially pathogenic bacteria. Sparkle might be introduced by aeration or by cascading water from one tank to another. The water was then distributed down earthenware, lead, or hollowed timber pipes. Earthenware was preferred as it provided better quality water, and was cheaper than lead, which even today can be found in piping in London. The Roman word for lead was *plumbus* hence plumbing, plumbers and plumb lines.

Wells and cisterns

Wells were an important alternative to aqueducts, especially for the home, with the advantage that the water was free, and hopefully 'on-site'. However wells are often found next to cess pits or rubbish dumps, since the Romans did not appreciate the dangers of ground water contamination. Although Pliny warned that water should come up from the bottom of the well, not enter through the sides, people were more concerned about getting clear and palatable water. Springs with clear mineral water often became the focus of a temple or healing shrine.

Rainwater was less well regarded, since it was flat and tasteless. However, physicians often used it as a basis for medicines – and possibly they realised that it produced less gastrointestinal disease than ground water from suspect sources. In drier parts of the empire runoff from the roof was collected in a cistern, and may have had to be used for drinking. Elsewhere it would have been used for decorative purposes in fountains and pools.

Drainage

Drainage was very important in Rome, for three reasons. First, the area was very marshy. The original drain, the *Cloaca maxima*, was said to have been constructed by Tarquinius Superbus in the sixth century BC, probably by alteration of an existing stream. It allowed Tarquinius to reclaim land for building the Roman Forum from the huge bogs that existed at the time. Three centuries later the drain was covered over, and is now connected to the city sewerage system. It must be the world's oldest functional sewer. The outlet is on the left side of the river just above the top bridge in Figure 2. The second reason for drainage was removal of the vast amount of water provided by the aqueducts, and finally there was flushing away the sewage of a million Romans. This was more to keep down the smell than anything else. Incidentally, when the Goths destroyed the aqueducts in 537 AD the city again became flooded and unhealthy. The Roman forum largely disappeared under the mud.

Baths and toilets

Before settling down to write this paragraph, I went to the health club – half an hour in the gym – then into the steam room and finally a swim. I suddenly thought – I'm doing just what the Romans did. Hippocrates had recommended hydrotherapy, but in addition, keeping fit and washing were regarded as important prophylactics against disease. Our pool is adorned by a statue – as were the baths in Rome, where Hygieia and Aesculapius figured large (second only to Venus and Bacchus).

The typical Roman would go to the baths daily after work. The bather would undress and be anointed with oil, then take half an hour's vigorous exercise (usually ball games) to induce a good sweat, helped by entering hot rooms. The sweat/oil would be removed using a scraper (Strigil), then a bath proper. The rich would be dried off, anointed with perfumes, then dress and go home. Bathing became a 'core function'. Baths grew bigger – often erected by rich men or emperors. The baths of Caracalla, which opened in 216AD, formed a sort of hypermarket with shops, restaurants, libraries and doctors on site, and covered 25 acres. They could accommodate 1,600 bathers at a time (6,000 per day). People would meet in the baths – dinner parties usually began there and continued at home.

Mineral waters were highly regarded for healing, as well as preventing illness. The spas at Bath and Buxton both have Roman origins. The King's Spring at Bath still produces nearly 300,000 gallons of water a day, full of minerals from beneath the Mendip hills and bubbling up at 46°C, no aqueducts required! Like other Roman towns, Bath later disappeared under the mud, and many of the buildings were pillaged for stone, especially for the cathedral and monastery built in the town.

However, the springs remained and were used for their medicinal properties until recently (see below). In 1790, when a new pump room was being built, workers found a Roman pavement 12 feet below the ground, and traces of a temple adjacent to the original bath. More exploration was undertaken a century later, when the Roman bath was restored, and the drain was followed backwards from the river Avon. Later major work including excavation of the temple is

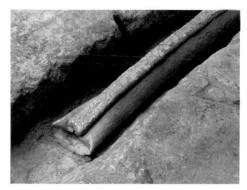

Figure 4   Lead pipe in the Roman Baths at Bath (Newsom)

as recent as 1970 and more remains are hidden under the Bath town centre. The main components of the Roman water supply are readily seen and include a lead pipe (Figure 4), the drain (Figure 5) (high enough to stand up in and still

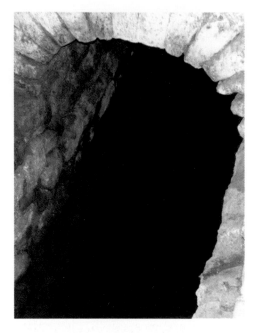

Figure 5   The main drain at Bath (Newsom)

working), and the bath – steaming and surrounded by the bases of the Roman pillars (Figure 6). The bath was lined with lead sheeting.

The abundance of water meant that most Roman baths had flushed latrines. Since many people lived in apartment blocks with no latrines, the communal ones were vital. There was more openness in their use than today. Many were multiple-seaters (Figure 7). Users would often chat or exchange dinner invitations while using the toilet. There was usually a water channel running around the room into which users would dip a sponge on a stick for use instead of toilet paper. Hence the expression: 'Getting hold of the wrong end

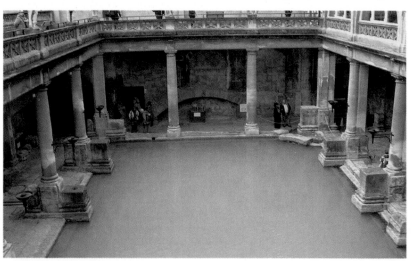

Figure 6   The Roman Baths at Bath (the colonnades are Victorian) (Newsom)

of the stick'. Public latrines also existed throughout the cities. Some had carved marble seats and statues. Only the larger villas had flushed latrines, which had to be on the ground floor, and were often sited in or beside the kitchen.

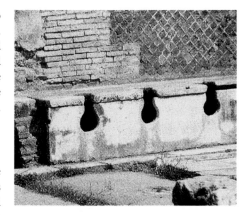

Personal hygiene

Since the causes of disease were largely unknown, great care was taken with personal hygiene and diet. Figure 8 shows a bronze Greek toilet set consisting of tweezers, toothpick, ear-scoop and nail cleaner found in Asia Minor, dating from around 300BC. Romans used similar sets, often carried around on brooches. In addition, the Romans used single silver toothpicks, or wooden ones made from the wood of the mastix tree (*Pistacia lentiscus* – often called the 'toothpick tree'). Toothpicks were popular gifts for dinner party hosts.

Figure 7   The latrines at Ostia

Teeth

Hippocrates discusses treatment for black gums and foetid breath: 'Burn the head of a hare and three mice, grind in a stone mortar then rub the teeth and all parts of the mouth'. Following

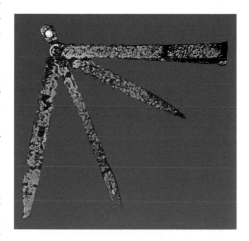

Figure 8   A Greek toilet set from 300BC

further medications, including anis, dill and myrrh dissolved in white wine, the teeth should become white and have a good smell. While this smacks of superstition, the charcoal produced by the burning is an effective agent. Later Roman recipes included hartshorn or hare head ashes as salves or mouth-washes, and Pliny described a toothpowder made from the burnt hoof of a goat. Then as now, shining white teeth were regarded as an asset. The Roman matron would have a slave girl – the *mastiche* – to lay out her mouthcare kit.

Diet

Nourishment was regarded as an important prophylactic against illness, while certain foods were regarded as cures. A specific example of the latter was the use of dock leaves for scurvy. Hippocrates had noted that scurvy followed a lack of fresh fruit and vegetables. The Roman army along the Dutch and north German coasts – well away from its citrus fruits was plagued by scurvy, but the tribesmen recommended *Radix britannica* infusions and these became an accepted treatment throughout the empire. The staple diet of the Romans however was grain – made into porridge, bread or pasta. This was supplemented by meat, fish and vegetables. In those pre-refrigeration days, the latter must have been eaten fresh. Romans liked lots of seasoning – coriander, fennel and garlic. One cook complained that 'cooks thrust herbs at you then season them with other herbs'. They had cookery books, and that by Apicius included medical advice.

Military hygiene

The Roman Empire depended on its armies, so as much care as possible was taken of the soldier's health. In fact, the army had a definite medical service, as did some cities – a classical predecessor of the NHS? New recruits underwent a medical examination. Physical fitness was monitored regularly: 'Those who are most knowledgeable in military matters', wrote Vegetius 'are of the opinion that daily exercise contributes greater health to soldiers than do physicians'. Equally important was basic hygiene. Although strategy dictated siting of camps and forts, wherever possible hygiene was also considered. Vegetius recommended: 'Do not keep the troops in … the vicinity of marshes, or arid plains'. Modern excavations reveal forts that were built on well-drained ground, usually adjacent to a river, which allowed a running water supply. Latrines were if possible of the stone-built flush variety and sewers emptied outside the camp, at best into rivers, and at worst into the surrounding ditch. If no running water was available a 'long drop' was used as a latrine, but needed cleaning out by the soldiers.

Large camps would have a hospital with the number of wards related to the number of soldiers, together with a surgeon, and possibly a physician. Hospitals were sited in a quiet area of the camp and usually had small rooms or wards, capable of housing a handful of patients (good for avoiding nosocomial infection). In addition, at least one large room seemed to be the operating theatre. This room usually had a fireplace for sterilising instruments or heating cauteries.

The downside

Despite the care that the Romans took, childhood mortality was horrendous, and of those who survived few working-class citizens lived beyond the age of 50; the wealthy (if not murdered) survived longer. An analysis of gravestones suggests that 28% of women and 38% of men reached the age of 62, a reflection of maternal mortality. Cemeteries were always sited outside city boundaries. The causes of disease were largely unknown, and contagion rarely suspected. Galen, a prominent Roman physician, referred to 'the seeds of disease', but what did this mean? Respiratory infections, including tuberculosis, were thought to spread between people, but poor air was thought largely to blame. There was no thought that human excreta were in any way dangerous, it was the smell that prompted their removal. Although food was necessary for good health, it was not normally thought of as bearing disease. One soldier wrote home complaining of acute food poisoning after eating rotten fish.

What of the baths? We have seen that these were used for keeping fit, but also for medicinal purposes. The emperor Hadrian reserved special bath times for the sick, but beforehand it was a free for all. Even the healthy must have stressed the system – they had sweated, scraped their skin, and been anointed before bathing (up to 6,000 in a day). Although many pools were fed with running water we have no idea how often the water was changed and of course there was no addition of chlorine.

Conclusion

Any attempt to be all-embracing of such a large topic at 2000 years' distance must be doomed to failure. However, I hope I have provided some food for thought on hygiene and infection issues before modern infection control had been established.

Postscript

A postscript to this occurred in Bath in 1979, when a girl died of infection with *Naegleri fowlerii* after bathing. Detailed investigations were unable to pinpoint and eradicate the source, and the Baths remain closed to bathers; protected with 'do not drink this water' warning notices. However, a new source of water is under investigation – so bathing in the Roman style may once again become possible.

Acknowledgement

I am grateful to Mary Ann Sullivan (www.bluffton.edu) for Figure 3.

Further reading

Cunliffe B. (2000) *Roman Bath discovered.* Tempus: Stroud.
Fagan GG. (1999) *Bathing in public in the Roman world.* Ann Arbor: University of Michigan Press.
Jackson R. (1988) *Doctors and disease in the Roman Empire.* British Museum Press: London.
Liversedge J. (1968) *Britain in the Roman Empire.* Routledge and Kegan Paul: London.

Chapter 12

Cholera part 1: John Snow and the beginnings of epidemiology

Introduction

Cholera used to be called 'Asiatic cholera', as it spread in waves (at least seven) from the Ganges valley, and differed from 'cholera morbus' – a milder diarrhoea thought to be due to excess 'choler' (bile). Like polio (Chapter 17), its reservoir is man, and spread is via the faecal-oral route.

However, the cholera vibrio survives in faeces and so can be spread by contaminated water and vectors such as the 'filthy feet of the faecal feeding flies'. With its acute diarrhoea, dehydration and 'rice water' stools, cholera has been known for centuries (Figure 1), but the first 'pandemic' to arrive in the UK came in the 1830s. It travelled slowly, coming by ship with infected sailors, and the effects were devastating.

The village of Upwell was struck down in 1832 by cholera from the neighbouring port of Wisbech. St Peter's church bears testimony to the disaster, which killed '63 people of all ages and either sex' within three months (Figure 2). The churchyard contains several mass graves marked with just a 'C' (Figure 3). Mercifully, cholera disappeared and did not reappear in the UK for 15 years.

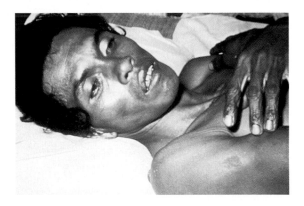

Figure 1   Cholera patient (CDC, Atlanta)

John Snow – early life

John Snow (Figure 4) was born in York in 1813. His father was a literate yet unskilled labourer, who nonetheless provided a basic education for his eight children. John was the eldest. At school he excelled in mathematics, and when he was 14 his parents 'apprenticed' him to an apothecary in Newcastle. He became a strict vegetarian and, like the rest of his family, teetotal.

He followed the ethos of John Frank Newton, who recommended that every family should have its own water distillation apparatus. Long before Snow's interest in cholera, drinking pure water was a dominant part of his lifestyle.

By 1836 he had become an assistant apothecary in the semi-inaccessible village of Pately Bridge. It was a dead end position, as he required a London qualification. So Snow moved to Soho, trained at the Westminster Hospital, and began a precarious living as a GP.

The London life allowed time for research. He studied neonatal asphyxia and respiration, and discussed his work with like-minded people at the weekly meetings of the Westminster Medical Society. Ten difficult years passed and he survived possible tuberculosis and kidney disease.

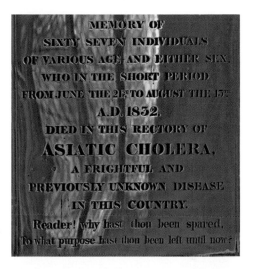

Figure 2   Memorial plaque at St Peter's Church, Upwell (Newsom)

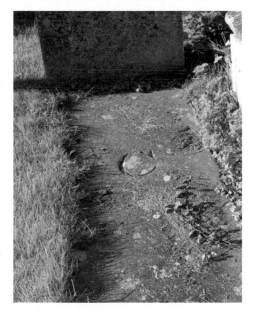

Figure 3   Cholera grave at St Peter's Churchyard (Newsom)

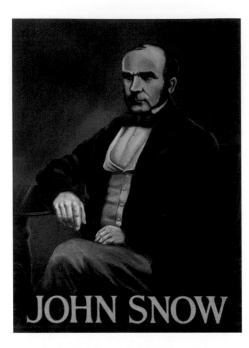

Figure 4   John Snow (inn sign) (Newsom)

Anaesthesia

Christmas week in 1846 was a defining moment both for Snow and for medicine. On Saturday 19 December, ether (first used by William Morton in Boston, USA two months earlier) was used for analgesia during a tooth extraction. Two days later Robert Liston, Professor of Surgery at University College Hospital, performed two operations under ether anaesthesia – one of which was attended by Joseph Lister, who was then a medical student. Liston said, 'This Yankee dodge, gentlemen, beats mesmerism hollow'.

On Monday 28 of December the dentist performed another operation 'in the presence of his friend Dr Snow'. Snow's life was transformed. He studied the effects of ether and invented ways to administer it, publishing regular bulletins in *The Lancet*. He became a successful anaesthetist, gave up his digs in Frith Street, and bought a house in Sackville Street.

The following year (1847), chloroform appeared. Snow inhaled some and found a pleasant inebriation, but thought nothing had changed until he realised the second hand had disappeared from his watch. Bulletins on ether were soon joined by those on chloroform.

The 1848 cholera epidemic

Cholera reappeared in London in 1848, and again in 1853. No one knew the cause, although it clearly had come from abroad. As late as 1853, an editorial in *The Lancet* said 'What is cholera? ...all is darkness, vague theory...' Two opposing theories were: 'contagion' (contact with a sick person's body or fomites) and 'miasma' (some vague atmospheric thing).

Treatment remained unaltered for years. Even in the spring of 1854 when Florence Nightingale was summoned to the Middlesex Hospital to nurse cholera patients she would have used traditional methods: turpentine poultices, chalk powder with opium, or brandy and laudanum. However, in 1848 an alternative treatment had been suggested: wrap in warm blankets, give a glass of brandy in hot water with sugar and spice, apply a poultice and place the patient under the influence of chloroform.

Snow would have known about using chloroform, although whether this triggered his interest is impossible to say. He had looked after patients in the 1832 epidemic. His writings thereafter had suggested he was a 'contagionist' and definitely against the medicinal use of alcohol.

The 1848 epidemic convinced him that cholera was a disease of the bowel, and was spread by faecal-oral transmission. Rather like Semmelweis (also in 1848) he postulated spread by microscopic morbid matter or particles and stressed the value of handwashing. His subsequent actions became a model for epidemiologists. First anecdotal experiences pointed the way, then a major point-source outbreak served to prove his hypothesis, and finally a retrospective survey showed how it all fitted.

Two reports by John Grant, the Assistant Surveyor for the Commission of Sewers came to Snow's attention in August 1849. The first involved Horseleydown by 'Bankside' in London's Southwark. Some five per cent of the Bankside population died of cholera in 1849, and four per cent in 1853. Originally they had disposed of 'nightsoil' in St George's fields and obtained drinking water from the Thames. However, the arrival of a piped water supply allowed for flushing toilets, and the fields were built on. As a result the Thames was now heavily polluted, so the value of piped water if obtained from the river was doubtful to say the least.

The first of Grant's reports was of a naturally controlled experiment in two adjacent blocks of houses (Surrey Court and Truscott's Buildings in Thomas Street). Between the blocks were privies and small cesspools, and beside them ran a polluted ditch.

Both were served with wells fed with water from the Thames by the same company. Initially people in both blocks developed cholera (presumably from the water), but thereafter only Surrey Court was affected (11 deaths compared to one in Truscott's Buildings). Grant found that the Surrey Court well often overflowed and water returned to the well contaminated with debris. The other well remained (relatively) clean.

Snow visited Southwark and noted: 'The surviving inhabitants nearly all left the place immediately after the above mortality occurred,' so he could not complete his investigation.

The other report concerned Albion Terrace in Lambeth ('genteel suburban dwellings of professional and tradespeople'), where initially one or two cases occurred.

However, an outbreak followed a heavy rainstorm, which presumably washed faecal matter into a drinking water tank. All the terrace tanks inter-communicated. When Grant went to investigate he found that one tank contained six to nine inches of deposit 'which possessed the odour of privy soil', some of which he sent to Snow. He reported 'on examination I found various substances which had passed through the alimentary canal, such as stones and husks of currants and grapes'. Altogether 20 people died and 'four or five were attacked after flying from the place'.

These two incidents led Snow to hypothesise that river water contaminated by cholera evacuations explained variations in mortality throughout London. He examined the weekly returns of births and deaths during the 1848 epidemic.

The data had been gathered by William Farr, the compiler of abstracts for the General Registry Office. Mortality south of the Thames, where water supplies came from the lower reaches of the Thames, was ten times that of the north, where clean water from other sources was used. This was no real proof, but was certainly a pointer. At least Snow noted that miasma was out – the smells in central London were no different from those south of the river. He published a pamphlet *The Mode of Communication of Cholera*. He later gave a paper and noted that pathology was confined to the gut, which had been poisoned by 'particulate matter' from faeces.

The London Epidemiological Society was founded in 1850. Snow and Farr were founder members. Snow was a regular attendee, although few members supported his cholera theories.

He was not unduly worried as his work on chloroform was prospering. He was asked to anaesthetise Queen Victoria during the birth of her eighth child in 1853. She 'appeared very cheerful and well, expressing herself much gratified with the effect of chloroform'. She was so pleased she demanded his services for her next delivery in 1857.

The Broad Street pump

The next cholera epidemic hit London in 1854. Snow studied water supplies and cholera south of the river, but his attention was soon diverted to nearby Broad Street. No such street exists today, as it became Broadwick Street in 1936. An old engraving shows the street as it must have been in Snow's day (Figure 5).

Originally this area to the east of Regent Street had contained houses for the rich, but by 1854 it had become apartments for the poor, sometimes four to five a room. In addition there was the Lion Brewery, the Eley Cartridge works, and a workhouse nearby.

On Monday 24 August, a Mrs Lewis, who lived at 40 Broad Street, washed her baby daughter's nappies in water, which she then emptied into the cesspool in front of the house. A few feet away people gathered around the water pump.

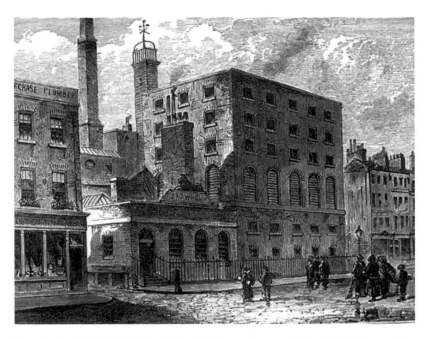

Figure 5   Broad Street in the 1800s with the Lion Brewery (pump was to the right of the brewery) (Old and New London, 1890)

The water was held in such high esteem that people came from neighbouring streets for it. The Eley brothers sent a daily flagon to their mother in Hampstead, and honoured their parent's wishes by keeping two barrels of fresh water in the factory.

No one realised that the baby had cholera. By the time she died on Saturday 'the angel of death had spread his wings over the place'. In the hospital Florence Nightingale noted that 'patients were brought in every half-hour from the Soho district, Broad Street …chiefly fallen women of the district'. She was up day and night attending to them. In the autumn she left for the Crimea well versed in cholera, which was already creating havoc in the armed forces there.

Cholera spared the people of Hampstead except for Susannah Eley, who died on Saturday, by which time several of the Eley factory workers were ailing. On Sunday Snow heard of the epidemic. As he knew that the north London water sources were unpolluted, he suspected a contaminated water pump.

He obtained samples of water from several pumps in the area. The Broad Street water looked the cleanest. However, microscopical examination revealed 'a good deal of organic matter' and some 'oval animalcules'.

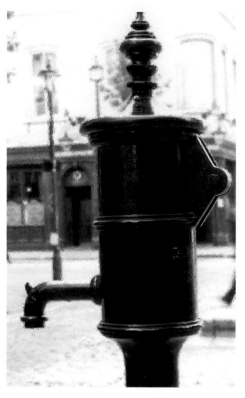

Figure 6 Broad Street pump (replica) (Newsom)

On Tuesday Snow obtained names and addresses listed on 83 death certificates from the registry office. He visited the relevant houses enquiring what water was drunk. He went to the surrounding areas and found that most of those affected had fetched their water from the Broad Street pump.

On Thursday he attended an outbreak meeting of the local Parish Board of Governors and Directors of the Poor and asked that the pump handle be removed. Although the board members favoured miasma as the cause, they nonetheless took Snow's advice (Figure 6). This was unpopular with the inhabitants who preferred the Broad Street water to their filthy water tanks. However, the epidemic subsided.

Snow later found that the number of deaths was much higher than he originally thought. Shoe leather was expended going round the area again, and in the end he produced a map relating cases to the Broad Street pump, and showing that in general people who used other pumps were unaffected (Figure 7).

Two other bits of 'negative data' supported his case. In contrast to the Eley factory where several workers died, there were no cases in the Lion Brewery, as the workers drank the beer. Furthermore, the workhouse had its own well, and so the inmates were spared.

Although the Board of Governors did not really believe the pump story they had it opened up and the brick shaft examined. It seemed perfectly in order. The cost of a cholera inquiry discouraged them from further action, but their consciences were assuaged when one of the most-involved clergymen, Henry Whitehead, curate of St Luke's church in Berwick Street, told them he could easily disprove Snow's theory.

Whitehead conducted a survey in February 1855, by which time the disease had died down, and he was able to take his time. However, far from damning Snow's hypothesis his survey showed in much greater depth that it was correct. Of those who drank pump water 58 per cent developed cholera, versus only seven per cent in those who did not.

He also found that the deaths related to people drinking the water in the first part of the period between the nappy-washing and the removal of the pump handle.

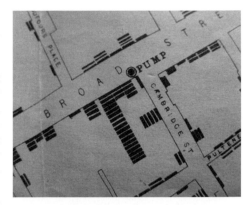

Figure 7   Extract from John Snow's map showing sites of cholera deaths and the position of the pump (NB The map is upside down compared to Figure 4 (Newsom)

He himself had had used pump water to dilute his brandy late during that dreadful week. This suggested that a 'pulse' of contamination had entered the pump shaft.

Another engineering survey was commissioned. This revealed that the cesspool drain was partially blocked and the earth between it and the pump shaft, which was only two feet eight inches away, was wet. The surveyors concluded that there had been a consistent leak from the cesspool to the pump shaft. Thus Snow's observations were fully substantiated.

In September 1855 the pump handle was finally replaced at the earnest request of the inhabitants, who still felt the quality of the water was much better than that in their own water tanks.

London's water supplies and cholera

Snow meanwhile continued to study death rates in relation to water supply using addresses of those who had died of cholera obtained from the registrar general's office. He concentrated on areas supplied by water from the Thames, which was becoming steadily more polluted.

Districts served by two companies, the Lambeth Water Company and S&V, had had equal numbers of cholera deaths in 1849. Both supplied water to the populations south of the Thames, sometimes to adjoining parishes. However, in 1852 the Lambeth water company moved its water intake upriver from Hungerford to Thames Ditton.

The two companies were in active competition. In many cases a single house had a supply different to those on either side. The experiment was on the grandest scale.

No fewer than 300,000 people of both sexes, every age and occupation, and of every rank and station were involved, and without their knowledge one group was being supplied with water containing the sewage of London.

The mortality in houses supplied by S&V water was eight to nine times greater than in those supplied by the Lambeth Water Company.

These results formed a major part of the second edition of *The Mode of Communication of Cholera*, which Snow issued in 1855. The book cost him £200 to print and he did not receive much return, either financial or scientific, for his money.

The present day value of a copy (if ever available) would be astronomic, but fortunately his papers were reprinted together with an introduction and biographical memoir in the 1930s (Figure 8).

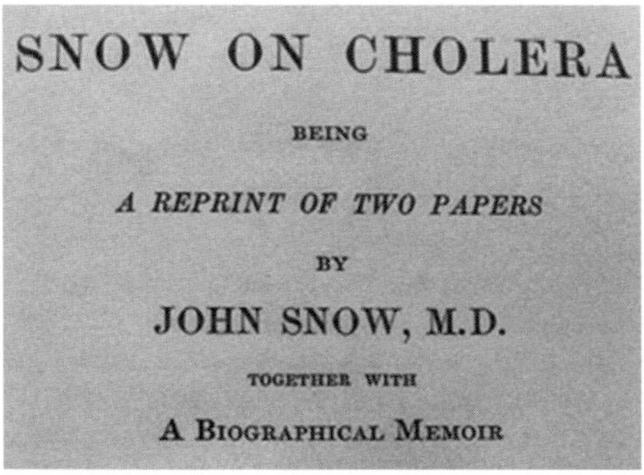

SNOW ON CHOLERA

BEING

A REPRINT OF TWO PAPERS

BY

JOHN SNOW, M.D.

TOGETHER WITH

A BIOGRAPHICAL MEMOIR

Figure 8   Snow on Cholera

Conclusion

The powers that be were slow to accept this work. Farr produced an amazing analysis showing that cholera mortality in London related to height above sea level and Sir John Simon (who became the first real medical officer of health for London) was also somewhat sceptical.

However, in due course both came to accept that Snow was right. Yet in the midst of his success he was struck down. On June 9 1858 he had just written the word 'exit' for his book on 'Chloroform and other anaesthetics' when he had a stroke – he died a week later.

1858 was also the year of 'The Big Stink' – such was the smell from the river that the curtains of the Houses of Parliament were soaked in chloride of lime. A bill was rushed through to provide a proper sewerage system. Thanks to a leading engineer Thomas Balgazette (see page 100), some 82 miles of 'sewage super-highway' were built with outfalls below the city. Cholera was finally conquered.

Much of the material from this article comes from a scholarly biography recently published by five professors from the Michigan State University (Vinten-Johansen et al, 2003). The breadth of Snow's work has made him one of the most revered scientists of his age. He pioneered 'geographical' epidemiology. The UCLA has devoted a website to his life and work (see www.ph.ucla.edu/epi/snow.html), while Broadwick Street contains the 'John

Snow' pub, with a first floor display devoted to his work (something his tee-total self might have disapproved of), and a replica of the famous pump.

The last word comes from a recent paper in *Public Health* (Bingham et al, 2004). The authors reworked Farr's data using logistic regression (a technique not available at the time) and showed that rather than the height above sea level, water supply was in fact the most important risk factor. Snow would have been pleased.

Further reading

Bingham P. Verlander NQ. Cheal MJ. (2004) John Snow, William Farr and the 1849 outbreak of cholera that affected London. *Public Health* **118**: 387–94.

Vinten-Johansen P. Brody H. Paneth N. Rachman P. Rip M. (2003) *Cholera, Chloroform, and the Science of Medicine. A life of John Snow.* Oxford University Press: Oxford.

Chapter 13
Cholera part 2: a continuing problem

Introduction

Snow observed that cholera was a 'poisoning' of the gut, spread by faecally-polluted water – possibly by 'particles'. However, even in London his work took time to sink in. My previous comment 'Cholera was finally conquered' referred to London and the sewerage system designed by Joseph (not Thomas – my thanks to a sharp-eyed reader) Balgazette. As we shall see cholera remains very much a feature of the 'global village'.

Later investigators, Koch included, seemed never to have heard of Snow's work. Nonetheless the current Mandell's *Principles and Practice of Infectious Diseases* concludes: 'Our understanding of cholera has improved since John Snow's day, but the solution remains the same.' Readers can find out more from the John Snow Society (see www.johnsnowsociety.org).

Pandemics seemed to start in the Ganges Delta – some thought due to emanations from the mud. However, there was no doubt that faeces were the key to spread, and were examined by the primitive microscopes available in the early 19th century. Fungal spores were found, but were also present in dysenteric stools. In 1847 Pouchet saw an 'extremely minute animalcule whose movements were rapid and sudden'; this was probably the first description of a cholera vibrio.

Rudyard Kipling's graphic descriptions of cholera in India have been published on the internet by Gillian Sheehan (see www.kipling.org.uk/rg_med_cholera. htm). 'Without the benefit of clergy' describes the spread of an epidemic: 'It struck at a pilgrim gathering of half a million at a sacred shrine. Many died at the feet of their God; the others broke and ran over the face of the land carrying the pestilence with them. It smote a walled city and killed 200 a day.' In 'At the end of the passage' the doctor says: 'And the worst of it is that the poor devils look at you as though you ought to save them. An old man was brought to me apparently beyond hope, and I gave him gin and Worcester sauce with cayenne. It cured him but I don't recommend it.'

Finding the vibrio

Epidemics continued to plague Europe, so in August 1883 when a new outbreak reached Egypt, Pasteur sent his assistants Roux and Thuillier to investigate. Franco-German rivalry was just as great as today, so the German government immediately sent out a team led by Robert Koch, fresh from his discovery of the tubercle bacillus (see Chapter 7). Within a week they had assembled an amazingly detailed travelling laboratory and departed. However, the Egyptian epidemic had abated by the time they arrived. The French team left empty-handed, but Thuillier died from cholera (the death was described in graphic detail by his colleagues). Koch's group failed to grow the bacteria or to infect animals – lack of fresh material was blamed. However, using his 'state of the art' microscopy, he was able to demonstrate 'comma bacilli' in autopsy material (see Figure 1). His report encouraged the German government to support an extension of his trip to India to continue his investigations. The *British Medical Journal (BMJ)* was doubtful – 'we hope should the results of the further investigations be negative, they will not hesitate to say so'.

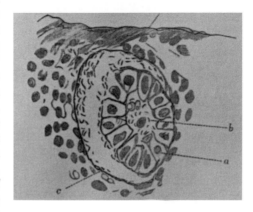

Figure 1　Robert Koch's drawing of cholera vibrios in the gut (Newsom)

The British authorities in Calcutta provided excellent facilities in the medical school, and there was no shortage of cases. A total of 42 autopsies and 32 samples of stools contained the bacilli. Within days the cholera vibrio had been grown in the laboratory, and even though one of Koch's own postulates – reproduction of the disease in animals – could not be fulfilled, the team were confident they had found the causative germ. Even the *BMJ* gave a grudging acceptance, but noted: 'It is by no means improbable, but quite possible that Koch's evidence may receive a wholly different interpretation by others.' Koch also showed how some cases related to a local water supply tank. This was also used for washing clothes, and contained viable cholera vibrios.

Koch made a triumphant return to Germany in April 1884. The bacteria had proved quite easy to grow, preferring a slightly alkaline culture medium. For many years alkaline peptone water was used as a selective medium; today a thiosulphate-citrate-bile salts agar is used and cholera vibrios give characteristically

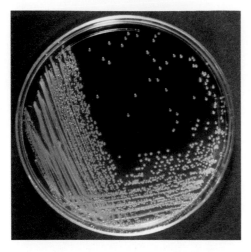

Figure 2   Cholera colonies growing on TCBS medium (CDC, Atlanta)

yellow colonies (see Figure 2). Sensibly Koch did not bring any cultures home as Europe was disease-free. However, later in the year cholera reappeared in France, and he readily isolated the bacteria from autopsy material in Marseilles. Even so, some remained unconvinced. Max von Pettenkofer was a celebrated hygienist in Munich who had a 'soil' theory – something in the soil was the problem. He thought cholera did not spread between humans, and water was irrelevant. He set out to prove that the cholera vibrio did not cause disease – he drank 1ml of broth containing around 10^5 vibrios. He was only mildly ill, unlike his poor assistant who also participated in the trial.

An epidemic in Hamburg in 1892 furthered Koch's cholera studies. These were published in 'Professor Koch on Cholera'. My copy (see Figure 3) of George Duncan's translation was given to the Hygiene Institute in Innsbruck by James Pollard of Edinburgh in 1894. Perhaps an English translation of a German book was an inappropriate gift – anyway to my surprise the pages were still uncut in 2005. Koch showed that infection in Hamburg related to water supplies. He made one important additional observation. The community of Altona was supplied with contaminated water from downstream of Hamburg. The water had filtered naturally through a bed of sand and the town was free of disease. He confirmed the value of sand filtration by laboratory tests. He also undertook another study on the geographic location of cases in relation to water supply, and while he makes no mention of Snow, he does refer to Farr's later work.

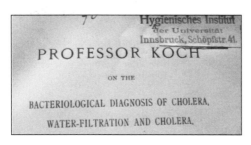

Figure 3   Koch on cholera (Newsom)

Pathology and prevention

Dehydration is a major feature of cholera. One of the earliest recorded uses of intravenous fluids was of a goose quill to allow venous access for rehydration. In 1953 De and Chatterjee (1961) showed that the pathology was due to the effect of a toxin (shades of Snow's poison) on the gut. They injected firstly whole cholera cultures, and later bacteria-free filtrates into isolated loops of rabbit gut. This laid down the basis for the World Health Organization (WHO) sponsored treatment of sugar and salt (from a two-ended spoon) dissolved in water.

By this time the cholera vibrios had been typed by agglutination tests with specific antisera. Two types (Inaba and Ogawa) were associated with full-blown disease, while a third type associated with a milder disease was called El Tor, after the Egyptian quarantine centre on the Sinai peninsular, used to isolate pilgrims who fell ill on the way to Mecca. On the other hand, non-agglutinable vibrios (NAGs) were not associated with disease.

Once Koch established that cholera was a bacterial infection, attempts to make vaccines began. The first vaccinations were made in Spain in 1885 by subcutaneous injections of a living culture. The side-effects were so bad that the government stopped further work. Pasteur's group also tried to make a living vaccine, but eventually killed vaccines were used. It was very difficult to evaluate these, because their introduction usually coincided with improvements in sanitation. Protection was assumed to be for a very short time – and cholera vaccination certificates for international travel lasted only for six months. Even in the 1940s, the British Army in Egypt confined soldiers to their camps rather than using the vaccine, which it was felt might lead to false confidence. Nonetheless vaccination became one of the mainstays of prevention.

Life in a cholera epidemic

The current cholera pandemic (the seventh) is due to an El Tor strain and started in Indonesia in 1961. At the time Hong Kong (HK) was an enclave of 400 square miles, containing around three million people. Many lived on junks moored closely together in harbours around the colony, or in shanty towns. Nonetheless there was a good water supply, and an organised health service. The Indonesian outbreak prompted a vaccination programme in March and April 1962, in which 53% of the population participated.

Cholera arrived in HK in August 1962. The first hint was that travellers from Canton showed roughly printed anti-epidemic certificates of inoculations against the four diseases (TAB, cholera). Then the press reported cholera in nearby Macau. The Director of the HK medical services (DMS) telephoned his opposite number in Macau, who denied the press report. Nonetheless an 'outbreak committee' was formed on 11 August to plan for an epidemic. The DMS's report

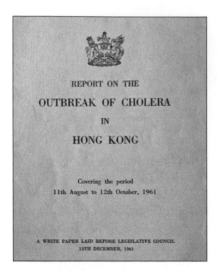

REPORT ON THE

OUTBREAK OF CHOLERA

IN

HONG KONG

Covering the period
11th August to 12th October, 1961

A WHITE PAPER LAID BEFORE LEGISLATIVE COUNCIL
13TH DECEMBER, 1961

Figure 4   Cholera in Hong Kong (PSI License C2009000939)

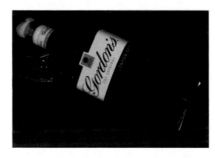

Figure 5   Cholera vaccine production (Newsom)

on the outbreak (see Figure 4) describes a model approach. The first things to be considered were isolation beds, a quarantine station, supplies of vaccine, provision of clean chlorinated water, disposal of rubbish/nightsoil (faeces), and institution of daily morning meetings. Mr Grimmo, the head technician in the government labs started a 24-hour vaccine production line. The supply of 'Roux bottles' normally used to grow the bacteria (shades of Pasteur) was inadequate, so the plea went out – Gordon's gin bottles please (see Figure 5).

Some 48 hours later, the DMS again phoned Macau to be told that one case had emerged. He sent a medical officer there on the afternoon ferry to take 10,000cc of vaccine and investigate. Canton and Macau were regarded as infected areas and all entrants from them were quarantined. On 15 August the first two cases appeared, so HK raised the 'yellow flag' and declared itself an 'infected area'. Health inspectors were diverted from inspecting houses to inspecting food, and mass vaccinations began. Rubbish disposal was monitored, and attention paid to general cleanliness (much improved) and 'the faecal feeding flies'. Because of the danger of leaky water pipes, chlorination was increased by 2.5 times, and chloride of lime was added to well water.

As the army pathologist my main role was to ensure that our laboratory had a fully functional cholera diagnostic service, and I visited the local mortuary to see autopsies on two cholera victims. Fortunately for me, no army personnel became infected. As a resident, the most obvious change was that cup of tea tasted of chlorine, and a bath was like a dip in a jacuzzi. Downtown long queues of people waited up to a whole day for their cholera jabs (see Figure 6) – good natured all the while.

I attended one outbreak committee meeting and was amazed at the range of items discussed, in particular relating to food – plans were made for the police to raid illegal food stalls the next morning, and the problems of overseas sales of 'moon cakes' much discussed. The mid-autumn festival was not far away, and HK exported 'moon cakes' to overseas Chinese throughout the world.

By 30 September the outbreak was declared over and the yellow flag lowered. In that time 61 cases had been treated in hospital and recovered, 15 died (eight in hospital, and seven brought in dead), and of the 731 contacts isolated, 53 grew the cholera vibrios. When one thinks of the population at risk, this was an amazingly successful exercise in outbreak control. The vaccination programme had involved giving two million doses – even Mr Grimmo's team working flat out could not provide that, but vaccine was donated from all over the world – the US providing 465,980ml (free).

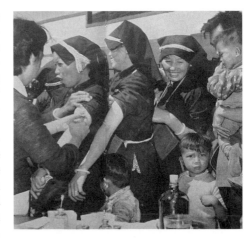

Figure 6   Vaccination under way (from Hong Kong Yearbook 1962) (PSI License C2009000939)

While HK had firmly raised the yellow flag, there was no information at all from China and we knew of cases in the Philippines. However, the authorities in Manila regarded their infections as 'El Tor disease', not cholera and refused to declare a state of infection. This was an early test for the WHO. The WHO Assembly had indeed passed a resolution in 1958 to the effect that 'infection with El Tor bacteria was not regarded as cholera for the purpose of international sanitary regulations'. However, the WHO regional centre made the Philippines see sense by holding an international meeting on the topic in Manila. Towards the end of September the Newsoms felt it safe to have a holiday in Japan. On arrival in Tokyo, no one was allowed off the aeroplane until all cholera vaccination certificates had been examined. To my great embarrassment, the customs examination of our hand baggage revealed one orange, which was promptly confiscated.

Spread of the seventh pandemic

The Newsoms came home in 1963 – by turbo-prop aircraft. The seventh pandemic took a much more leisurely route, and finally arrived in Europe (Portugal) in 1977 (see Figure 7). In the 1980s it moved to Africa, and crossed to South America in the 1990s. Indeed 745,560 cases occurred in South

America in 1991 to 1992. The latest WHO record is for 2004, when 94% of the cases were reported from Africa (95,000). So unlike its predecessors, the seventh pandemic has persisted and indeed cholera has merited a chapter in a recent book on 'emerging infections' entitled *New challenges from a once and future pathogen* (Scheld et al. 1998).

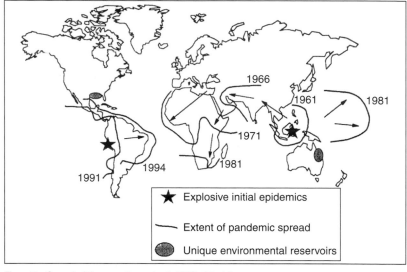

Figure 7   Spread of the seventh pandemic (CDC, Atlanta)

Several human factors have contributed to this persistence. Mobility has increased. When we left Kai Tak airport to come home, there might have been 16 intercontinental flights a day landing in HK. Today it will be one every two minutes. Goods continue to be shipped around the world, and ships often discharge water ballast near land. Finally expansion of the human population and its concentration in cities outstrips the provision of water and sewerage systems. Even as I write (in January 2006), ten cases of cholera including three deaths have been attributed to poor maintenance of the Harare water supply. (By 2009, Zimbabwe was undergoing a full-scale outbreak involving thousands of cases.)

Conclusion

Snow's work raised several questions that have now been answered. Firstly the Broad Street baby was a prototype. We now know that babies can be a good source of bacteria, often without being ill. Secondly he showed that 60% of people who used the Broad Street pump became infected. What of the others who did not? Why was Pettenkofer able to drink the culture (albeit a strain of low virulence)? We now know that the vibrio likes an alkaline medium. Recent work has shown that infection with *Helicobacter pylori*, which causes hypochlorhydria in the stomach increases the risk of acquiring severe cholera (Clemens et al. 1995).

Finally what about the mud? Snow had reported sludge in the 'privy soil' in Albion Terrace. The work of Colwell and Huq (1994) started from the observation that Bangladeshis could develop cholera even when it could not be cultured from the water. They thought that the bacteria might be dormant (non-culturable) – unable to grow on culture media, but possibly 'switched on' when in the human gut. This proved to be the case. Dormant bacteria can be demonstrated by staining with fluorescent antibodies, and it turns out they are often associated with tiny crustaceans called 'copepods'. Up to 10,000 vibrios can adhere to a copepod, which is found in brackish water and lives on plankton and algae.

In contrast to polio, cholera vaccination has had only limited application, with the killed-cell vaccine producing perhaps a 60% protection rate, lasting only a few months. Clearly more work is required – and newer vaccines are in prospect. They may well be needed as global warming increases the population of algae, and encourages the copepods.

Further reading

Clemens J. Albert MJ. Rao M. (1995) Impact of infection by *H. pylori* on the risk and severity of endemic cholera. *J Infect Dis* **171**: 1653.

Colwell RR. Huq A. (1994) *Vibrios in the environment: viable but nonculturable Vibrio cholerae:* In: Wachsmuth IK. Blake PA. Olsvik O. (Eds.). *Vibrio cholerae and cholera*. ASM Press: Washington DC: 117–33.

De SN. (1961) *Cholera*. Oliver and Boyd: London.

Newsom SWB. (2006) John Snow, Henry Whitehead, the Broad Street pump, and the beginnings of geographical epidemiology. *Journal of Hospital Infection*. **64**: 210–216.

Scheld WM. Craig WA. Hughes JM. (Eds.). (1998) *Emerging infections*. ASM Press: Washington DC.

Chapter 14
Legionnaires disease part 1: the Philadelphia outbreak

Introduction

The American Legion (Figure 1) is an organisation of veterans of the US armed forces, founded after the Great War in 1919. It has around 3 million members and organises remembrance and other events, and is politically active. Local 'Posts' are grouped into State 'Departments.' 1976 was a special year, marking 200 years of American independence, and the Pennsylvania Department of the Legion arranged a major convention lasting from 21–24 July, with balls, dinners, meetings and a parade. Around 4000 members and guests were involved. The meeting was centred at what was originally one of the most luxurious hotels in the world – the Bellevue Stratford (B-S); built on the main street (Broad Street) of Philadelphia in the early 1900s (Figure 2). However the convention became dogged by an epidemic of pneumonia, in which 221 people, mainly delegates, were involved and 34 died. Not all were legionnaires – some had only walked past the hotel or witnessed the parade on Broad Street, and for a time the 'Broad Street' pneumonia existed, but was soon merged into the 'Legionnaires' disease.

Although the causes of community-acquired pneumonia had gradually been revealed when fastidious germs like *Mycoplasma pneumoniae* and *Chlamydia psittaci* became cultivable, some

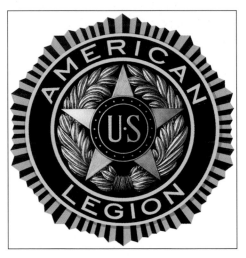

Figure 1   The American Legion (Newsom)

cases remained inexplicable. My father's dictum 'it must be a virus', for unknown infections certainly applied here to begin with.

Like typhoid and cholera (shades of John Snow) Legionnaires disease is waterborne. The causative organism presents several paradoxes – it is difficult to grow in the laboratory, but naturally widespread in water and water supplies. The disease is largely man made – both from modern sources for infection such as cooling towers, complex building water supplies, showers etc, and because we have a susceptible population including smokers, senior citizens, and hospital patients (particularly the immunosuppressed). Although epidemics create a great public awareness of Legionnaires disease 65–75% of infections are

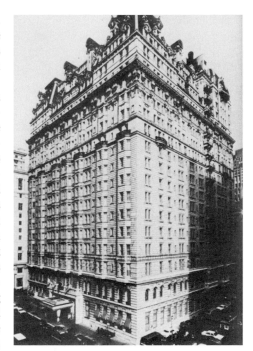

Figure 2   The Bellevue Stratford Hotel

sporadic, some of which are nosocomial. It is probably under-diagnosed and under-reported so 18,000–88,000 cases per year are thought to occur in the US. *Legionella* research is very much ongoing and still justifies regular international conferences.

The Legionnaires' outbreak

The issue of the *New England Journal of Medicine (NEJM)* for 1st December, 1977 is unique; it contained reports of the outbreak and the isolation of the causative organism (Fraser et al. 1977; McDade et al. 1977) together with an editorial (Figure 3). Gordon Thomas and Max Morgan-Witts interviewed those mainly involved in the outbreak and wove their results into *Trauma* (1981) – a modern thriller that just happens to be true (Figure 4). The two publications complement each other and provide a clear account of the outbreak. The progress of the investigation was followed in a series of reports in the CDC newsletter – *the Mortality and Morbidity Weekly Report (MMWR)* (Sharrar and Parkin, 1976; Anon, 1997).

Six hundred and twenty-two Legionnaires and families checked into the B-S on Wednesday 21 July. This was the headquarters hotel – with lectures and hospitality suites, and in the evening a remembrance service was held in the ballroom for 1000 delegates. Delegates were largely housed in three additional hotels, but came to the B-S for functions. The lobby was always crowded. Legionnaires brought in their own beer (to the hotel's annoyance) and although 30% of those questioned never drank water in the hotel, the use of ice exceeded capacity and extra supplies had to be shipped in. Later a taxi driver found his car boot being dismantled by the police – but no potential ice contaminants were found.

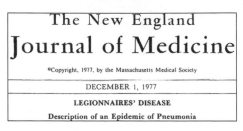

Figure 3   *The New England Journal of Medicine* article (Fraser et al, 1977)

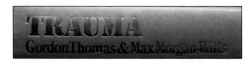

Figure 4   A thriller!

Afterwards people recalled some unhappy omens. The city refuse collectors were on strike, pigeons (Figure 5) were everywhere, and despite the cold war, Tall ships from Russia were moored at the jetty for the centennial celebrations. In the B-S lobby, a man in a shiny blue suit (not a legionnaire) was heard to say, 'it is too late – you will not be saved'.

The climax of the event was a parade, passing down Broad Street on Friday. Many were bussed in for the event – one bus driver watched, like many others, from the pavement in front of the B-S, and members of one band ended by marching into the ballroom. However by now several delegates were 'under the weather.' The legionnaires then dispersed across the state.

The disease spreads

A week later there were signs of trouble; 72 people were ill, and two had died. The legionnaire's conference organiser was told of the deaths – but felt they were not out of the way for such an elderly population. A doctor in Williamsport reported to the public health authorities that three legionnaires had presumed typhoid, and the infection control nurse from Chambersburg Hospital reported three who had pneumonia, one of whom died. Both got the same response – nothing can be done until Monday!! Nonetheless the Philadelphia epidemiologist, Dr Sharrar, was contacted at home on Saturday by a doctor from Carlisle, who reported a case of *mycoplasma* pneumonia, and said he had heard of other cases of pneumonia from Philadelphia, including a death in Lewisburg. Sharrar reacted immediately – it sounded as though his main fear was being realised – an outbreak of swine influenza – similar to that which had claimed thousands of lives in 1919. There had already been national discussions on vaccination – but not enough vaccine was available. Sharrar telephoned the Lewisburg pathologist, who confirmed that the patient had died of a viral pneumonia; so he asked for samples of tissue to be sent to the State microbiology laboratories in Harrisburg, the State capital.

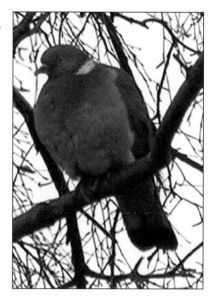

Figure 5   A red herring (Newsom)

Investigation commences

By Sunday five legionnaires were in hospital in Williamsport. The post commander visited them, and was told that the only positive culture was *klebsiella* from one sample of sputum. He was concerned enough to contact the State Health Department, and on Monday things began to move. The Communicable Disease Center (CDC) in Atlanta was contacted by a doctor from Philadelphia who reported 11 deaths, and gave a possible diagnosis of swine flu. However because the CDC was a national organisation, it could not move without an invitation from the State Health Department. This was soon forthcoming. A press conference had been held in Harrisburg, by which time the media knew of 12 deaths and 40 cases in hospital – they swarmed over the B-S. Media suggestions included plague, Lassa fever, and bioterrorism (not a word much used then). However the CDC felt that influenza was likely, and so dispatched a 'swine flu' team, headed by Dr David Fraser.

On Tuesday, when Fraser arrived in Harrisburg, he was told of 100 patients, with 19 deaths – a horrendous mortality. The number of new cases reported was declining, however, and there was no evidence of secondary cases, which minimised the possibility of influenza. Nonetheless, later antibody tests revealed flu antibodies – but this elderly population would have been involved in the 1919 pandemic. By now other cases had emerged: the bus driver who had watched the parade, ten members of the band, a truck driver delivering meat to the hotel, and a clerk working in a bank across the road. Food, air, or water seemed likely routes for infection – but if air – why had none of the hotel staff been affected?

What about bioterrorism? The US biological warfare unit at Fort Detrick, was not far away, but had ceased functioning ten years earlier. However a military truck with an FD registration was seen to be parked near the parade route. Had it leaked germs or toxins? It was never explained away. Fraser developed questionnaires for the legionnaires, and thanks to their organisation, 3,683 were completed. He also had 32 'leg men' from CDC gathering data. Public health nurses were asked to search hospitals for legionnaire patients. A 'hot line' was set up and the public asked to report suspected cases. Case control surveys were set up.

CDC was now providing laboratory back-up. One hundred scientists began work on toxicology, tissue from autopsies, and sera. Some 30 metallic elements were looked for (especially paraquat), and cultures set up for 77 known infectious agents.

By Thursday 5 August questionnaires were ready for distribution, and the State labs confirmed that negative cultures in eggs ruled out influenza. A report appeared in the *MMWR*, with Sharrar as the first author. Autopsies had suggested an 'interstitial' pneumonia suggestive of a viral origin, and so material was sent to the CDC. Meanwhile a CDC expert in buildings, George Mallison, was checking out the B-S. He found the kitchens in good order, crawled around air supply ducts, and inspected water supplies and refrigeration. A dead pigeon in one duct suggested psittacosis, and there were some cross connections in the plumbing, of unknown significance. The lobby staff also reported that the air conditioning outlet was blocked, and the main cooler kept leaking refrigerant. One unexplained clue was the repair man who went off sick with respiratory infection, for which he took some tetracycline, and whose family were also sick. He refused to give any blood samples, possibly another red herring.

Later Fraser moved to Philadelphia, and housed his team in the B-S (making them guinea pigs). Analysis of questionnaires from hospitalised patients revealed that 39 (two deaths) were **not** legionnaires. They had not visited the B-S, but all had been within one block of the hotel, and so were labelled 'Broad Street Pneumonia'; six others had stayed in the B-S attending the Eucharistic conference that followed the legionnaires meeting (Figure 6). Person to person spread was finally ruled out. By 22 August all local investigations were complete, and the CDC team returned home to analyse the results. However the B-S had received a fatal blow – by the end of September only 10% of beds were occupied, and so the hotel was shut down.

Finding an agent

At the CDC, influenza, typhoid, and many other bacterial diseases were soon ruled out. No known pathogen grew and serology was negative. Joseph McDade

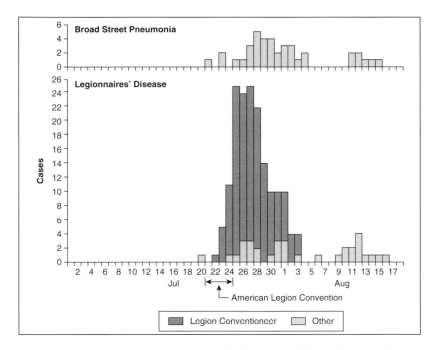

Figure 6   Progress of the epidemic (from *The New England Journal of Medicine* Fraser et al, 1977)

was asked by his boss Charles Shepard to make cultures for coxiella (Q fever) or other rickettsiae, as being 'hard to grow' 'incomplete' bacteria.

According to *Trauma* McDade drew a blank. He inoculated guinea pigs with material from four postmortem lungs, and demonstrated a rising temperature within 1–2 days. However when he subcultured guinea pig material into eggs, there was no reaction. His serology was negative, and after six weeks he gave up. Enter Dr Sheila Katz, who was a pathologist in Philadelphia. Some days after doing a 'legionnaires' autopsy she developed a chest infection. She treated it with tetracycline and recovered. However she later did some electron microscopy on her sputum and saw 'mycoplasma-like, pebble-shaped' forms. She visited CDC, but was not taken seriously – but in fact might well have been on the right track.

Again quoting from *Trauma:* On 27 December, for reasons he was never clear about, McDade had another look at tissue from his infected guinea pigs. This time he could see intracellular bacteria. He then succeeded in growing the *legionella* in eggs – the embryos died in 4–6 days. The reason for the previous failure was that using virological techniques he had added antibiotics to his material before infecting the eggs!!! None of this is reported in the *NEJM.* Proof that this was the cause of the pneumonias was soon provided by demonstrating antibodies in 91% of patient's sera using indirect fluorescent antibody tests. Interestingly only one of the hotel staff tested (a cashier) had antibodies, but no clinical symptoms. Presumably this was because they were young and healthy!

Conclusion

The investigation of this outbreak represents an epidemiological triumph worthy of John Snow, complemented by discovery of the causative organism. The CDC had had to work in an ambience of unprecedented media interest. There had been daily 'body counts,' more rumours of biological and chemical warfare, and accusations of a 'cover-up' by the CDC. When the first results came out, Shepard and McDade were all for publication in a peer-reviewed journal, but the political scene required immediate reaction. So a compromise was reached – the *MMWR* is a scientific publication, and the announcement was made in a special MMWR supplement on 18 January, 1977, one day after the initial positive tests on tissue from two patients had been repeated once (in the first extra issue of the MMWR ever published). In accord with the disease, the organism was called *Legionella pneumophila*, but it was soon joined by *Legionella micdadei*.

The source of the outbreak was never conclusively found – not surprising as the causative organism was unknown at the time. However, the mode of spread was thought to be through the air. By the time the articles appeared in the *NEJM,* retrospective studies showed that previous outbreaks – in a mental hospital in Washington, and a Health Headquarters building in Pontiac were also due to *legionella,* of which several different types and serotypes were now discovered. The message had got out already, and in November the *Lancet* carried details of the first cases in Europe – UK holidaymakers from Spain, whose sera was shown to contain antibodies at the CDC (Lawson et al., 1977). Later when cultures became practicable, my colleagues in Cambridge (Nagington et al. 1979) made some of the first isolations in Europe (while many of their colleagues were away in Atlanta, attending the first international *legionella* conference), and also found a new serotype. Several outbreaks have occurred in healthcare premises in the UK, and I became involved in water testing – especially after infections occurred in our transplant patients. But that is another story.

Further reading

Anon. (1997) From the 18 January 1977, special issue of *MMWR*. Epidemiologic notes and reports follow-up on respiratory illness – Philadelphia. *Morbidity and Mortality Weekly Review* **46(03)**: 50–6.

Fraser DW. Tsai TR. Orenstein W. Parkin WE. Beecham HJ. Sharrar RG. Harris J. Mallison GF. Martin SM. McDade JE. Shepard CC. Brachman PS. (1977) Legionnaires' disease. *New England Journal of Medicine* **297**: 1189–97.

Lawson JH. Grist NR. Reid D. Wilson TS. (1977) Legionnaires disease. *Lancet* **ii**: 1083.

McDade JE. Shepard CC. Fraser DW. Tsai TR. Redus MA. Dowdle WR. (1977) Legionnaires' disease. Isolation of a bacterium and demonstration of its role in other respiratory disease. *New England Journal of Medicine* **297**: 1197–203.

Nagington J. Smith D. Wreghitt T. (1978) Isolation of Legionnaire's disease organism in Cambridge. *Lancet* **ii**: 1144–5.

Sharrar RG. Parkin WE. (1976) Respiratory infection – Pennsylvania. *Morbidity and Mortality Weekly Review* **25**: 244. (5 August 1976).

Thomas G. Morgan-Witts M. (1981) *Trauma*. Hamish Hamilton: London.

Chapter 15

Legionnaire's Disease part 2: Outbreaks and errors

The last 30 years has seen the development of knowledge about *legionella*; how the disease is spread, and its therapy. Unlike other water-borne microbes *legionella* appear naturally in water, and are spread to humans via aerosols. Most infections are sporadic, but outbreaks such as those in the UK at Kingston and Stafford Hospitals hit the headlines. The dangers of recycling hot water and wet cooling systems have become apparent, and the need for a high index of suspicion and quick response to finding unexpected cases – as in transplant patients in hospital or linked cases such as two BBC workers on one day – is essential.

Introduction

The previous chapter described the 'Broad Street Pneumonia', and ended with Joseph McDade growing *legionella* at his second attempt, by inoculating guinea pigs followed by egg-yolk cultures. Enough antigen was produced to demonstrate antibodies in sera from the sufferers. Although the original bacterial cultures were negative, by the time the seminal paper of McDade et al (1977) was published, cultures on a Mueller Hinton agar enriched with haemoglobin and yeast extract had been successful, so providing material for a diagnostic fluorescent antibody test. However the source of the epidemic remains a mystery.

Today we know of 49 species of *legionella*, half of which can infect humans. *Legionella pneumophila* serogroup 1, the cause of the Philadelphia outbreak, accounts for more than 70% of human infections. They are unusual bacteria (Figure 1) – using protein rather than carbohydrate as an energy source, and they grow best on a buffered charcoal yeast extract agar containing l-cysteine (BYCE) at 20–40°C, growing slowly so that detection of antigen in a patient's urine is the quickest reliable diagnostic test.

Legionnaire's Disease is water-borne like cholera and typhoid, but the bacteria appear in water as a result of natural rather than human pollution, and infection is a result of inhalation of an aerosol, rather than ingestion. Just as cholera vibrios live inside copepods, *legionella* can live and multiply into large numbers inside amoebae, which may form cysts and protect the bacteria from the environment, especially when in bio-films. There is also a dormant 'sporelike' form of *legionella* with enhanced resistance that is hard to detect. The main danger for humans is man-made, coming from the complex water supplies and cooling systems required for large buildings. Blind loops, stagnation, and the siting of hot and cold water pipes side by side are all potential hazards.

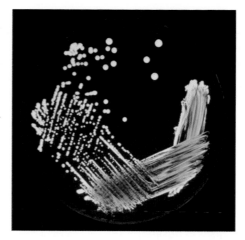

Figure 1   Fluorescent colonies of legionella (Aquagard Ltd)

Although outbreaks of Legionnaire's Disease hit the headlines, 75% or more of infections are sporadic and account for 2% of all patients with pneumonia requiring treatment in hospital. A community-wide study suggests that 18,000–80,000 cases occur annually in the USA. The main sufferers are elderly people, although those with immuno-suppression are also at risk. Hospitals as large buildings with complex water supplies housing susceptible patients are thus high-risk areas. McDade et al's (1977) paper included positive serology from patients in a psychiatric hospital where an unsolved outbreak of pneumonia had involved 81 cases with 12 deaths.

I am going to review the outbreaks in Kingston and Stafford Hospitals and the one that affected Broadcasting House in London, describe my own involvement in diagnosis and research, and finally comment on the recent outbreak in Barrow-in-Furness.

Kingston Hospital – 1976

By 1976 Kingston Hospital had a new seven-storey building (Fischer-Hoch et al, 1981). Between December 1979 and July 1980 12 cases of Legionnaire's disease occurred. Eight were in patients with other illnesses housed in the new building (five on the top floor), two were hospital staff, and one was a visitor. The last patient had pneumonia following a holiday in Spain (already a recognised risk factor). In June 1980 an outbreak was suspected. The cooling-tower sited on the roof was found to be contaminated with *legionella*. It was cleaned and chlorinated, but although samples became negative four more cases occurred and the water was once again found to be contaminated. Despite twice-weekly chlorination, residual chlorine levels soon dropped off, and in November the tower was abandoned.

Three more infections diverted attention to water supplies. The main supply entering the building was negative, but hot and cold water from taps throughout the new building grew *legionella* as did the holding tanks in the roof. So the somewhat Draconian measures of adding extra chlorine to the water main, and recirculating hot water at 55–60° were instituted, and the outbreak ceased. However despite these precautions a further case occurred a year later. This time *legionella* were found in the hot water supply, and traced to the heat exchangers (claorifiers), one of which had been turned off although it remained connected to the hot water circuit (Fischer-Hoch et al. 1982).

Papworth Hospital – 1985

Early in 1985 a patient recovering from a heart transplant developed pneumonia with *L pneumoniae* serogroup 5. The experts were called in and found the same *legionella* in the calorifiers and in the hot water system, including the showers used by the transplant patients. The main water tank and cold water storage tanks were free from *legionella* but grew other aquatic organisms. As at Kingston we found that one of the calorifiers had been switched off, although remaining connected to the hot water supply which was recycling (Figure 2). The water contained 9.3×10^4 *legionella* per litre – consistent with counts found in other outbreaks.

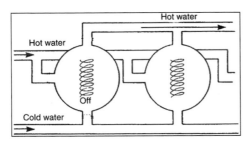

Figure 2   Diagram of Papworth hot water supply with left hand heat exchanger switched off, but remaining in the circuit (Newsom)

By now suspicion had also pointed to flexible shower pipes and washers inside shower heads, and indeed water samples from the two showers in the transplant suite had similar counts to that in the calorifier – higher than those in the hot water generally. The showers were dismantled, and with due warning the hot water in the system was raised to a temperature of around 80°C (at the taps) at 8pm one evening, then the system was drained and a hearty hour spent in gumboots cleaning out the main water tanks on the hospital roof (mainly of sand), before adding chlorine and flushing the system with the chlorinated water. The last line of the protocol

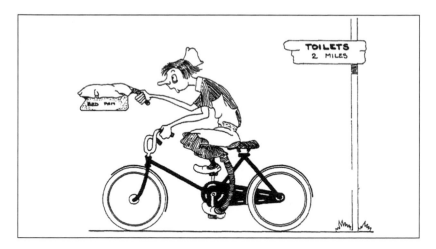

Figure 3   Planning plumbing (HMSO, PSI License C2009000939)

read: 'for Dr Newsom to carry out the necessary tests on the following day!' By now I had learnt the technology, and the tests, done by filtration of a 5 litre sample were negative.

Stafford – 1985
In the early 1970s when Legionnaire's Disease was unknown, I was a member of a Department of Health Planning Group concerned with Public Health Engineering. One of our projects was design of the 'Harness' hospital. This turned out to be too expensive and only two were built; it was supplanted by the cheaper 'Best Buy' design. Fortunately for my peace of mind our role was only concerned with drainage (Figure 3). The design was based on a grid, and in the centre of each cross piece was a roof-mounted cooling tower. The new 'Harness' hospital in Stafford was opened in 1983. The cooling towers provided a novel challenge to the hospital engineers, the more so because tower 4 serviced the air conditioning for some high-dependency units as well as the outpatients, and although *legionella* had been grown from it in November 1984 it was not shut down for the regular maintenance recommended by the Department of Health in 1980 after the Kingston outbreak.

In April 1985, 101 people (mainly outpatients) were admitted with a pneumonia that turned out to be Legionnaire's Disease, and 28 died (the largest outbreak since Philadelphia). Most of them had only visited the hospital once, and in fact the last patient became infected *before* the first case of pneumonia was admitted, and the source of infection disappeared as mysteriously as it had arisen. Establishing the diagnosis took some time and highlighted problems with the infection control structure. The infection control technician post had been discontinued in March, the consultant microbiologist was much involved in a neighbouring hospital, and the trainee was on holiday. The consultant physicians faced with 10 new cases a day asked for help from the Birmingham virology department, where a tentative diagnosis of influenza was made. The local laboratory staff, being unaware of any urgency, sent samples to Manchester by post, which were then transferred to Preston. Thus it took at least 10 days to establish the diagnosis.

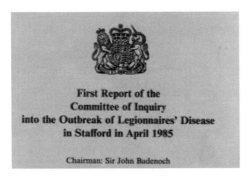

First Report of the
Committee of Inquiry
into the Outbreak of Legionnaires' Disease
in Stafford in April 1985

Chairman: Sir John Badenoch

Figure 4   The Badenoch report (HMSO, PSI License C2009000939)

The gravity of the outbreak warranted a Committee of Inquiry, which was chaired by Sir John Badenoch and reported in June 1986 (Figure 4; Badenoch report, 1986). This highlighted the need for proper infection control services, and a 'major outbreak plan'. An in-depth investigation of water supplies and drains was undertaken, and the probable cause of the outbreak was a design fault, complicated by inadequate maintenance. The air inlet for the ventilation system was only 3 inches below that for cooling tower 4, and immediately below its exhaust. A marker gas released at the air intake of the cooling tower could be detected in the Outpatient Department, having passed through the tower and then down into the air conditioning intake (see Figure 5).

Cambridge 1986–90
The Stafford outbreak prompted a great interest in keeping cooling towers *legionella*-free. Hinchingbrooke Hospital had a cooling tower that was well maintained and carefully monitored. A large volume of air passed through the water being cooled, and any particulate matter was washed out and ended as dirt in the cooling tower pond. So when I was asked to test an 'ultraviolet steriliser' I was a little suspicious because although UV irradiation can be used to sterilise water, the water has to be clean. Anyway the system was installed in the Hinchingbrooke tower, and the result surprised even me – after a few weeks the whole thing became completely blocked by algae, which had been stimulated by the ultraviolet.

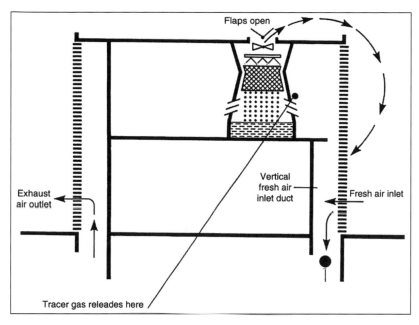

Figure 5   The Stafford cooling tower showing how near the building the ventilation inlet was sited (3 inches) (from Badenoch report, HMSO, PSI License C2009000939)

Soon after the Stafford incident Barney Hayhoe, the Minister of Health, was asked: 'So what is the future for water cooling in the NHS', 'None at all,' came the reply.

Meanwhile another transplant patient – this time in Addenbrooke's Hospital turned up with Legionnaire's Disease. The 10-storey building presented a much more complex problem than Papworth. However I went into the basement to the calorifiers (at last I realised why the wards above were always so hot), and took a 5-litre sample of water. The pressure from the tanks 10 storeys above was so high that the minute I opened the tap – I got a shower. When the sample grew a moderate growth of *legionella*, I became worried, but I was much younger then and remained healthy. However what to do with the hospital's hot water? This time there were no blind loops or turned off calorifiers, so we repeated the turning up the heat in the middle of the night, and went round opening hot taps. Fortunately this worked, and the problem disappeared, although I suspect it is very difficult to maintain a *legionella*-free situation.

By now *legionella* worries had spread into the community and I was asked to test water from a fountain in the centre of a shopping arcade (no problem); but

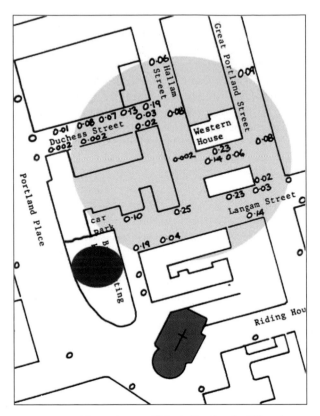

Figure 6   The BBC map. Brown = All Souls Church, red = BBC, and
pink = approximate area contaminated by spray from the cooling tower
(adapted from City of Westminster Report: Cunningham, 1988)

potentially more worrying – from the humidifying mist in the greenhouses of the botanic garden. If anything was a good and potentially infectious aerosol this was it – and although visitors were kept out during the spraying, they entered soon afterwards. Anyway all was well, cultures were negative, but for a time I was worried.

Broadcasting House – 1988

The BBC outbreak in Portland Place, while not hospital-associated, forms a good contrast to that in Stafford (Cunningham, 1988). It also related to a rooftop cooling tower, and involved 79 cases, only 70 of whom were ill, and two died. The lesser morbidity and mortality reflected the at-risk population – healthy and younger people rather than hospital patients, together with prompt therapy. The diagnosis was made much sooner than that in Stafford because the two initial cases were seen at an infectious disease unit (in Romford) on the same day (27 April), and samples were sent on 29 April by taxi directly to a laboratory (in Chelmsford) with a 2-hour turnaround time. The physicians found that both patients, although living in different areas, worked at the BBC, and so they immediately informed the Communicable Disease Surveillance Centre and the city health departments. The Chelmsford public health labs remained on stand-by despite the bank holiday weekend.

The investigators had the Badenoch report available and immediately formed an outbreak control committee. The BBC engineers were told to switch off the cooling towers, but to wait for sampling before decontaminating them, and indeed the next day large numbers of *legionella* were demonstrated directly in the water from one tower; both towers were then treated. Many people walked past the BBC building daily, and several surrounding buildings had cooling towers and so a major case-finding exercise was required – all the intensive care wards in London were contacted, and the BBC itself publicised the problem. After 10 days there were no new cases and the epidemiology pointed to a single source outbreak on April 21/2. The weather – high humidity and a light SW wind would account for the at-risk zone, and later tests with tracer gas inserted into the B cooling tower inlet on a similar day showed detectable levels of gas in the streets below. Indeed the map (Figure 6) reminds one of that produced by John Snow for the cholera cases only 1.5 km away in Broadwick Street. The offending tower was removed soon afterwards.

Conclusion

By the 1990s the epidemiology of *legionella* was well worked out, and in addition to Department of Health advice to hospitals, the Health and Safety Executive updated protocols for protection in 2001. The 2002 outbreak affecting 180 people with seven deaths in Barrow-in-Furness (Health and Safety Executive, 2007) therefore came as a surprise. The answer was human error – 'In summary there were a number of mistakes made by different officers over a period of time, all of which, contributed to the outbreak' (Health and Safety Executive, 2007) – a perennial problem.

Like polio, Legionnaire's Disease can be regarded as a result of civilisation – in this case related to complex water supplies, rather than better sewage. Unlike polio and typhoid where the main reservoir is human – *legionella* are everywhere and so legionellosis can be expected to continue. Although routine sampling of normal water supplies is unrewarding, it has been recommended for transplant units. A single hospital-acquired case of Legionnaire's should ring an alarm bell.

Civilisation can bring unexpected problems – like the day I found balls of black fungi and worms in the water from tanks in *two* supermarkets – but that is another story (Newsom, 1999)!

Further reading

'Badenoch report.' First Report of the Committee of Inquiry into the outbreak of Legionnaires Disease in Stafford in April 1985. Chairman: Sir John Badenoch. (1986) London: Her Majesty's Stationery Office.

Cunningham D. (1988) Broadcasting House Legionnaires Disease; report of the Westminster Action Committee Environment Committee, Westminster City Council: London.

Fischer-Hoch SP. Bartlett CLR. Tobin JO'H et al. (1981) Investigation and control of an outbreak of legionnaires disease in a district general hospital. *Lancet*: 932–6

Fischer-Hoch SP. Smith MG. Colbourne JS. (1982) Legionella pneumophila in hospital hot water cylinders. *Lancet* **i**: 1073.

Health and Safety Executive. (2007) Report on the Public Meetings into the legionella outbreak in Barrow-in-Furness, August 2002. (2007) http://www.hse.gov.uk/legionnaires/barrow.htm Accessed 5 Jan 2009.

McDade JE. Shepard CC. Fraser DW. Tsai TR. Redus M. Dowdle WR. and the laboratory investigation team. (1977) Legionnaire's disease: isolation of a bacterium. *New England Journal of Medicine* **297**: 1197–203.

Newsom SWB. (1999) Black pigmented fungi in water. *Journal of Hospital Infection* **41**: 254.

Chapter 16

Typhoid fever: another a continuing problem

Introduction

Typhoid or enteric fever has been known for centuries – although the final stages of the illness (the typhoid state) are almost indistinguishable from those of typhus fever, another scourge of the ancient world.

The Emperor Augustus who as we saw (in Chapter 11) was cured by his Greek doctor (Antonius Musa) was said to have had typhoid. Queen Victoria's husband Albert was among many notables who died of the disease. The clinical picture of epidemic typhoid was documented by Thomas Willis (better known for describing the 'circle of Willis' formed by cerebral blood vessels) in 1659.

The worldwide incidence is estimated at least six million cases, with 600,000 deaths a year – mainly in Africa and Asia. In 2005, an epidemic in the Congo involved 42,500 cases with 214 deaths. Like polio and cholera, it is a strictly human infection, and spread via the faecal-oral route. The Commu-

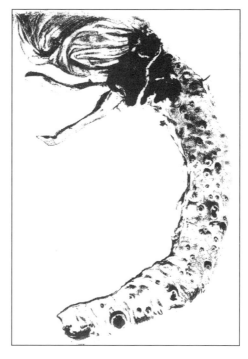

Figure 1   Typical ulcers of small bowel (Budd, 1873)

nicable Disease Surveillance Centre (CDSC) recorded only 248 cases in England and Wales in 2006, 122 of which were imported, reflecting the value of good sanitation (recently awarded the most important advance in health since 1840 by readers of the *British Medical Journal* – out of 15 'medical milestones'). Such improvements are within living memory as my grandmother died of typhoid in 1940.

My interest in the epidemiology was sparked off in 1946, when by chance we drove through Aberystwyth on the very day an outbreak started – spread by ice cream. Luckily for me, we didn't stop, but my description of the outbreak contributed to a distinction in my school certificate exams.

The reservoir of infection is the human carrier (a word first used by Robert Koch – typhusbazillentrgerin). Carriers may have recovered from the disease, or be entirely 'silent'. Carriage can persist for ages. Four senior officers planning the D-Day invasion of France in 1944 who went to stay at a pub in a remote Devon village caught typhoid. The organism was of an unusual type, last seen in the Boer War 40 years earlier. Investigation revealed a veteran of that war living nearby, and sewage from his house entered an open drain that passed in front of the pub.

The most famous carrier was Mary Mellon, immortalised in *The Ballad of Typhoid Mary* (see later). Carriers can excrete large numbers of bacilli – one in Islington produced enough to be detected at the north London sewage outfall.

Bacteriology

The bacteria were first described in 1880 by Joseph Eberth, a German pathologist working in Halle, in intestinal ulcers seen at post mortem. They were grown in pure culture from the spleens of 40 typhoid victims by Dr Gaffky working in Koch's laboratory in Berlin in 1884.

A few years later, Koch's team produced a 'selective medium', which allowed typhoid bacteria to grow, while other faecal bacteria were suppressed. However they were unable to fulfil 'Koch's postulates', in that they could not infect an animal with the cultures (Gaffky, 1884).

Originally called *Eberthella typhosus*, the name rapidly changed to *Bacillus typhosus* (the organisms were rod-shaped), and later when gram-negative bacilli were re-named *Bacterium*, it became *Bacterium typhosum*.

In the late 1930s, it became clear that there was a large group of similar organisms (2000 or more), which were called *Salmonella* in honour of Daniel Salmon, a US veterinary bacteriologist who worked on them in the late 1880s. During my working life, we had *Salmonella typhi*. Now molecular methods have further subdivided the salmonellas, and we have *Salmonella enteritica var typhi* as a cumbersome but accurate name.

Salmonellas are very robust, and unlike similar organisms such as *Escherichia coli*, they resist desiccation and survive well on surfaces. *S. typhi* differs from other salmonellas both *in vitro*, and *in vivo*. The bacterial cells have some metabolic differences, and a thick polysaccharide capsule – called the Vi(rulence) antigen. Unlike other salmonellas, which are widespread among animals, infectivity is strictly limited to humans, and the disease produced is systemic. Recently the genetics have been analysed in depth, and S. *typhi* was found to lack some normal salmonella genes.

The infecting dose for S. *typhi* is relatively low, and this combined with its resistance means that typhoid (like cholera) is one of the few diseases spread by water. The bacteria can multiply in food – which is clearly another major route of spread.

Clinical picture

The bacteria are ingested. While small numbers may be killed by acid in the gastric juice, those that escape find a haven in the duodenum, being stimulated to grow by the bile (often used in bacterial culture media).

The incubation period is around ten days while the bacteria multiply in the gut and are filtered through the 'Peyers patches' (collections of lymphoid cells) into the blood stream causing a gram-negative septicaemia. The fever climbs in a 'stepladder' manner, and is remittent, allowing it to be separated from the 'intermittent' fever of malaria, or the 'undulant' fever of brucellosis. Two unusual features are the pulse rate that does not climb in parallel with the fever (relative bradycardia), and neutropenia.

Another sign of infection is the appearance of 'rose spots' caused by bacteria settling in the skin capillaries. During the third week of illness, the bacteria have settled again in the Peyers patches, and cause ulcers in the gut wall. The two most lethal complications of these are perforation and haemorrhage.

Untreated, at least 10% of patients will die, and in the over 60s and under threes mortality may be 50%. The 'typhoid state' (confused with typhus) is of a patient lying on his back, too weak to move, unconscious of his surroundings, his trembling

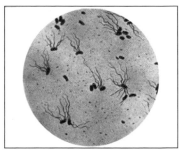

Figure 2 *Salmonella typhi* – stained to show flagella (CDC, Atlanta)

hands picking aimlessly at the bedclothes, his eyes deceptively bright but seeing nothing – to be followed by the deep coma and the death rattle. Recovery is often accompanied by less severe relapses, and many become carriers with bacteria persisting either in the gall bladder (sometimes causing cholecystitis) and being excreted in the faeces, or in the kidneys being excreted in urine.

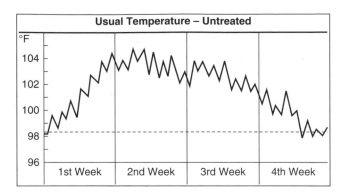

Figure 3   Typical temperature chart (Huckstep, 1972)

Good nursing remains the mainstay of therapy. Gut complications can be corrected by surgery. Specific therapy only became available with the introduction of chloramphenicol in 1949 – a toxic and not too effective drug (patients still had relapses). The quinolones such as ciprofloxacin and gatifloxacin are much more effective, although quinolone-resistance is becoming a problem.

Epidemiology

William Budd, working in North Tawton, a village north of Dartmoor where he grew up, first documented an epidemic of typhoid among the villagers in 1839, well before the germ theory of infection. He noted the seriousness: 'No one can ever know what it implies, who has not had experience of the fever in his own home. The dreary and painful night-watches... The long suspense between hope and fear... and the large number of cases in which hope is disappointed and fear realised...'

His book (Budd, 1873) is a masterpiece of microbiological detective work (before bacteria were discovered!). He followed the disease through families and to neighbouring villages – for example two carpenters left the village already ill, and started new epidemics. He insisted it was contagious and spread by contamination of milk and water, and emphasised the dangers of excretions from a convalescent patient. He noted that the villagers had no running water or drains, and their cesspits were dangerously close to their wells.

Amid other outbreaks he describes was one among 140 people who attended two Balls held two days apart in a hotel in Cowbridge. He discovered that a visitor to the hotel had gone down with typhoid shortly beforehand and the cesspool was so near the well used to make drinks (such as lemonade) for the dancers, as to make percolation from the one to the other inevitable (shades of John Snow, Budd indeed also studied cholera).

Even before this James Chadwick, a lawyer had championed sanitation – he felt that infections spread by contaminated air from drains were a major cause of loss of earnings and poverty, and involved much government expenditure on 'poor relief'.

He recommended piped water for flushing the drains. Even so many years passed before proper water supplies and sewage were provided (shades of the 'Great Stink' of the 1850s). By 1900, only 40% of people in Holland had piped water, and 50% had access to sewers, and the UK was in a similar state.

An outbreak of typhoid (around 3000 cases), which occurred in Gelsenkirchen in 1901, was described by Howard-Jones with the subheadings of 'Robert Koch and the dead hand of Max von Pettenkofer' (Howard-Jones, 1973). This outbreak occurred because at times of water shortage, untreated river water was mixed in with the normal supply. The waterworks was prosecuted for purveying foodstuffs injurious to health. Koch was the main prosecution witness, while Pettenkofer's succes-

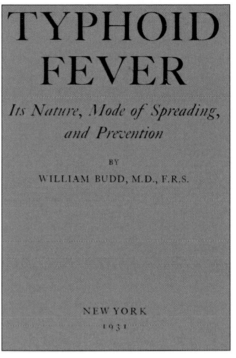

Figure 4   Budd's book (reprinted)

sor in Munich, Emmerich, gave evidence for the defence – noting the theory that typhoid bacteria were harmless by themselves, and needed 'maturation, before being spread through the air'. Koch won out, but it was some years before Pettenkofer's theories (including that on cholera) could be finally laid to rest.

Two later epidemics illustrate the dangers of complacency even when proper hygiene is in use. Firstly is the Croydon epidemic of 1937 (Murphy, 1938), which claimed 43 lives and involved over 300 cases of typhoid.

At the time one-sixth of the town water came from a deep well in the chalk at Addington. The well was being cleaned out, and one of the workmen was a typhoid carrier. The men were lowered into the well on a plank, accompanied by an open bucket to avoid having to be lifted out to urinate.

The suggestion is that the bucket was not used. As the raw well water had been repeatedly tested and shown to be pure, the water treatment plant was closed for maintenance. There was doubt as to who was responsible, but both the filtration and the chlorination were turned off. Certainly the plant engineers had no idea that the well was being cleaned at the same time.

The second outbreak which occurred in Aberdeen in 1964 (Special correspondent, 1964) was the first to be subjected to the modern media treatment. Over 500 people were affected, and Aberdeen became 'a beleaguered city', and warranted a morale boosting visit from the Queen.

The epidemic was traced to a 6 lb tin of Argentinian corned beef, being sold by the slice in a local supermarket. Careful detective work traced the victims back to the supermarket, although not all had bought beef. One was a vegetarian. At its peak over 50 patients a day were being admitted to hospital with suspected typhoid. All from one tin of beef? The beef slicing machine had acted as a secondary source.

Corned beef is by its nature cooked, and *S. typhi* is not unusually heat resistant. However, an inspection of the canning factory in the Argentine, revealed that the cans were cooled in river water. As they cooled, temporary leaks opened and closed in the seals. Even so how could the salmonellas multiply, when they are strictly aerobic bacteria, and the sealed tin would be free from oxygen. A clever bit of detective work by Peter Meers showed that the sodium nitrite used in processing could act as a 'hydrogen acceptor' and so allow the bacteria to grow.

This was the last major typhoid outbreak in the UK, and it certainly had repercussions in the area of food safety. Today other Salmonellas occupy our thoughts – particularly *S. enteritidis*, and eggs. Interestingly enough this is one of the few other Salmonellas that can cause systemic disease, although it rarely does so.

Mary Mellon

A recent biography of 'typhoid Mary' was published by Anthony Bourdain, himself a chef (God sent us meat, but the devil sends us cooks) (Bourdain, 2005). Mary was born in Ireland in the 1870s and became a cook employed by wealthy families in New York in the early 1900s – her *forte* was peach ice cream.

She had several jobs as people always kept getting ill from her cooking – 35 known cases were traced to her, but she may well have been responsible for over 1000. When the Warren family fell ill in their rented vacation house on Long

Island, the owner, fearing that the house would become unlettable, employed Dr George Soper – a sanitary engineer to check it out.

The only unusual finding was that they had employed a new cook three weeks before the first illness, and she had left without comment after the third person had become ill. Soper turned himself into a detective – cooks for wealthy families usually came from two or three employment agencies, so he could trace Mary – and unearthed other families with typhoid.

When he found her and tried to interview her she fled, and when the city authorities finally acted it took three policemen to arrest her. Eventually she was 'exiled' to a hospital on North Brother Island in New York. However, four years later (1910), she was released 'having learnt her lesson'. Not so.

Hospital-acquired typhoid

The main danger in hospitals is the undetected carrier. However an epidemic occurred in the St Lawrence State Hospital in 1903, due to use of ice from the St Lawrence River. No one would have drunk the water, but the ice (kept in an ice-house until the summer) was supposed to be germ-free.

Typhoid also has a bad reputation with laboratory workers. Over 250 cases of typhoid have been laboratory acquired, largely due to handling suspensions of the bacteria, so that today it is categorised as a dangerous germ requiring special handling facilities.

Within a year of starting in laboratory medicine, I was involved in typing an isolate of S.typhi using slide agglutination. In my eagerness, I breathed too closely on the slide and swallowed some bacteria. A hasty oral toilet followed by pro-phylactic chlorampenicol saved the day.

In 1915 there was an outbreak of typhoid among the staff of the Sloane Hospital for women in New York. The servants had jokingly named the cook Typhoid Mary. Soper claims credit for being called in and recognising Mary's handwriting – however it is certain that like other staff she had a stool culture, and by the time the typhoid bacilli were grown she had vanished. However, she was eventually traced by the authorities and made to return to her exile permanently. She finally made a reasonable living as a laboratory technician, and lived until 1937.

A recent episode involved our own hospital head cook, who caught typhoid while on a Middle East holiday. While incubating the disease, she went on a union-sponsored bus trip for a weekend in Germany. Blood cultures were found to be positive on a Saturday afternoon – our technician had been taught of the dangers of typhoid, but thought she was dealing with a normal E. coli bacteraemia.

When I told her what she had grown (I had done some quick typing tests), she had to be revived with cups of tea (nothing stronger available). Anyway a

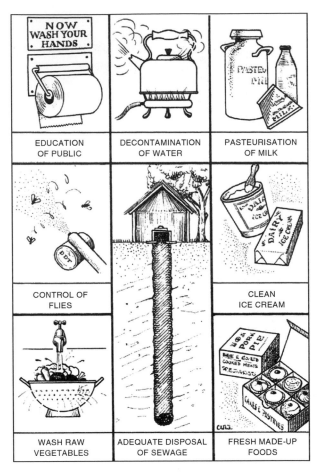

Figure 5   Prophylactic measures (Huckstep, 1972)

'warn the GPs to look for unexpected fever in recently hospitalised patients' went into action, but no secondary cases occurred.

Prevention

In the Boer war in South Africa the English army lost 8,000 men to typhoid – this is often called 'The last of the typhoid campaigns'. Certainly the army took a great interest in water hygiene and in typhoid vaccines thereafter.

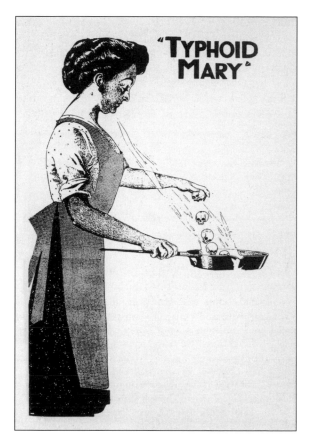

Figure 6   The most famous typhoid carrier (Mary Evans Picture Library)

The first vaccines made by heat treatment of whole cells were made only a few years after Gaffky grew the bacteria. The army medical services consumed 50 million cubic centimetres of typhoid vaccine in World War I. So although ten times as many soldiers were involved, only 1191 died of typhoid. However, this is not as easy as it seems – much of the improvement could have been due to better hygiene.

Certainly a major problem in testing typhoid vaccines has been that any community in which they are tested may well have improved the sanitation during the test making it meaningless. What to actually use for the vaccine has been a major bone of controversy over the years, especially since the discovery of the Vi antigen in 1932.

Whole cell vaccines containing lipopolysaccharides can cause fever – indeed the vaccine was used as a cure for syphilis in the hopes that a fever would allow the body to kill the spirochaetes. My last injection – given in our army hospital in Malaya gave me a temperature of 40°C and the worry that I had caught malaria.

More recently a purified polysaccharide vaccine containing the Vi antigen has been used. An oral vaccine is also available. These certainly are painless, but their efficacy is nothing like as good as for example oral polio vaccine.

Conclusion

Typhoid fever has a vast literature, and I have only skated the surface with items of personal interest. The book written by RL Huckstep in 1962 when he was a surgeon in Kenya makes for good well-illustrated reading.

As typhoid is a purely human condition, it should, like smallpox and polio, be possible to eradicate it completely. However, although in developed countries the disease is gradually disappearing as the unsuspected typhoid carriers die out and proper sanitation prevents new cases, in the developing world there is clearly a long way to go.

Further reading

Bourdain A. (2005) *Typhoid Mary.* Bloomsbury Press: London.

Budd W. (1873) *Typhoid fever: its nature, mode of spread and prevention.* Reprinted by Public Health in America. (1931) Arno Press: New York.

Gaffky G. (1884) 'On the etiology of enteric fever'. Reprinted in: *Recent essays on bacteria in relation to disease.* (1886) New Sydenham Society: London.

Howard-Jones N. (1973) Gelsenkirchen typhoid epidemic of 1901:

Robert Koch and the dead hand of Max von Pettenkofer. *British Medical Journal* i: 103–5.

Huckstep RL. (1962) *Typhoid fever.* E&S Livingstone: Edinburgh and London.

Chapter 17

Poliomyelitis part 1: Ancient Egypt to 1950 – a disease uncontrolled

Introduction

Polio normally only affects humans and so, like smallpox, there is a hope of banishing it from the world. The World Health Organization reported 1263 cases for the year until March 2005. Most of these cases (789) occurred in Nigeria and a lesser number (189 cases) were on the Indian subcontinent.

In the UK infections are rare and follow polio vaccination. This was not the case when I was young. Annual epidemics frequently occurred in the late summer and in the US a record 60,000 cases occurred in 1952.

I well remember going to bed with a fever in the autumn of 1947 and our doctor testing my reflexes daily, while my anxious parents looked on. In 1949 our school was closed for two weeks by another outbreak. Two boys died and everyone was sent home, while the school captain of athletics became wheelchair-bound. It is no surprise then that I have had a lifelong interest in polio, and the controversies surrounding the vaccines. Indeed, my first publication in 1959 (Figure 1) was on the topic.

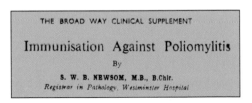

THE BROAD WAY CLINICAL SUPPLEMENT

Immunisation Against Poliomylitis

By

S. W. B. NEWSOM, M.B., B.Chir.

Registrar in Pathology, Westminster Hospital

Figure 1   My first publication (1959)

Unlike smallpox, the definition of polio as a disease and the discovery of its cause was a gradual process. 'Club foot' was documented in Egyptian times (Figure 2), possibly the very first depiction of any disease. Only later was it recognised that a 'teething fever' in babies was sometimes accompanied by paralysis, and the name of 'infantile paralysis' appeared. The author Paul de Kruif called it 'the maiming death'.

In the 1800s autopsy studies confirmed the clinical impression that this was a disease of motor nerves – sensation was not affected. The pathologists showed that the 'grey matter' (or to be specific the anterior horn cells) of the spinal

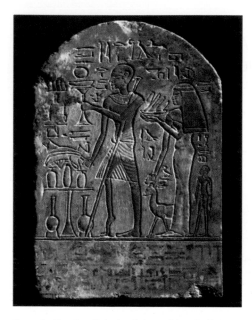

Figure 2   Egyptian Stele showing possible polio victim (Wikipedia)

cord were involved. This gave rise to the name 'poliomyelitis' from Greek words meaning 'grey' and 'matter' followed by the Roman 'itis' meaning inflammation.

Although Koch had shown how to grow bacteria, none could be found in these patients, and it was left to Karl Landsteiner and his assistant Dr Popper in Vienna in 1908 to prove that a virus was involved. They did this by injecting monkeys with a filtrate from the spinal cord of a polio victim. The filtrate had already been cultured for bacteria and shown to be harmless to mice, rabbits and guinea pigs. They could only afford two monkeys (Landsteiner was a pathologist in a general hospital), but this was enough to show that the disease was due to a virus.

Having provided a major landmark, it is a pity they could not afford to continue their research. However, we owe much more to Landsteiner because he defined the A,B,O blood groups, and was rewarded with a Nobel prize for immunology.

Epidemiology

Polio is a disease of civilisation. In the past the viruses clearly saturated the human population, babies were infected within six months of birth and so would have been protected by their mother's antibodies. Few clinical cases occurred.

The virus is transmitted by faeces, and as sanitation improved babies were no longer infected. A susceptible population developed, and epidemics occurred, mainly among older children and young adults.

The earliest properly documented epidemics occurred in Sweden between 1885 and 1911, where doctors observed that the disease was contagious and that in an epidemic some children developed the same feverish illness without becoming paralysed, but the virus could be isolated from them. They also showed that virus could be isolated from naso-gastric washings and faeces, although the significance of these findings was not recognised for many years.

Soon afterwards the main focus moved to the US. The New York epidemic of 1916 was the worst then on record (7,000 cases) and remained so for many years. Paul De Kruif spelt it out in graphic terms: 'That hot summer in New York one child out of 80 was struck with the paralytic peril… one morning a mother would go into the room of her baby to find the child could not move its arms or legs, or couldn't talk or swallow or breathe properly.'

Public health officials enforced a draconian quarantine on affected families, but it was to no avail. They concluded that the disease only affected humans, but the presence of many subclinical cases and carriers made quarantine useless. Carriers became immune to reinfection, like those recovering from the disease.

Other clues and blind alleys occurred. Tonsillectomy seemed to encourage paralysis. Using monkey spinal cord to make a vaccine (shades of Pasteur and rabies) failed, as did the use of antiserum from monkeys or convalescent children.

The cost of animals limited polio research. However, both the Rockefeller Institute and Yale University set up research teams. By 1934 things were not much further forward, and so when an outbreak occurred in Los Angeles there was panic and the 'experts' from the east were summoned.

The experts set off by train (a four-day trip) accompanied by 50 monkeys. Dr Webster's letters to his wife set the scene: 'A telegram was received asking we get off the train at Pasadena to avoid the crowd waiting for us at the terminal. They said the mayor was waiting to meet us and give us the freedom of the city... We actually met his brother as he had been called to quell a riot. Then the press – 15 reporters and 10 cameras.' They had expected a team from Yale to be in blazers and boaters, not scruffy scientists. 'Pictures were taken and then they shouted "now for the monkeys". "Nothing doing" said we. "What's the matter Doc, ain't you going to give us a break?" But we were adamant. As for the epidemic, 50 cases a day admitted to hospital – 20 of the nurses in charge and four doctors down – one after another.'

The team worked very hard, but only recovered the virus from two patients. A total of 2,499 people were suspected of having polio, but it seemed as though not all were genuine – a case of mass hysteria, perhaps.

Red herrings

In the early 1930s two American doctors tried again to make vaccines. There was a great competitive pressure, for whoever succeeded would become a national hero.

The only source of virus was still infected monkeys, but both doctors felt that 'stock strains' of virus that had been passed from monkey to monkey were stable enough to use as a basis. Dr Brodie went for an emulsion of monkey spinal cord that had been treated with formalin to inactivate the virus (on the lines of diphtheria immunisation), while Dr Kolmer produced a living, but tamed virus – he called it 'attenuated'. Both reported success in monkeys, and later in humans. There was no Food and Drugs Admistration then – Brodie inoculated 3,000 children after safety tests on only 20 monkeys. Kolmer tested his product on 42 monkeys, but had at least used himself as the first human to be vaccinated.

When the Kolmer vaccine was used on 10,000 children, 10 caught polio from it. Both vaccines were severely criticised and neither were heard of again. Ten years later when an eminent scientist suggested to a national meeting that 'The time has come to find out what happens in man' (when vaccinated) it is reported that 'a veritable shudder went around the room, and the subject was immediately changed'. Indeed, this was such an unhappy experience that it was 15 years before any further attempts to make a vaccine.

Another 'preventive measure' tried was the nasal antiseptic barrier. The Swedish work on spread via faeces had not been followed up, partly because it was almost impossible to decontaminate them so monkeys developed brain abscesses from intracerebral injections.

However, virus had been found in nasal washings. Was it spread through the air like influenza? Early tests on monkeys had shown that they could be infected by swabbing their noses with virus. The nerve endings in the 'cribriform plate' at the top of the nose connect directly to the brain – scientists wondered if this could be the portal of entry for the virus (Figure 3), and therefore if it could be blocked.

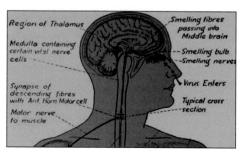

Figure 3   A possible passage of virus – justification for the 'blockade'

In 1937 when Paul de Kruif wrote his book blockade seemed the most hopeful approach. Swabbing monkeys' noses with alum before challenging them with the virus did indeed prevent infection. In the words of the book: 'In one cage lies a monkey who is limp and powerless. He is no longer full of monkey merriment. Beside each wrecked beast, scampering, romping screaming... is an absolutely healthy monkey.'

However, when investigators poured alum into their own noses, 'it caused a most infernal tickling, stinging, sneezing and then a dryness lasting several hours'. Picric acid was less irritant, but a new problem arose. The human nose differed from the monkeys and it required an ear, nose and throat surgeon to accurately cover the 'cribriform plate' with the chemical. Occasional trials were made before the whole idea was dropped as impractical.

Franklin D Roosevelt

The most famous and also the most actively supportive polio patient was Franklin D Roosevelt, who became the longest-serving president of the US despite being paralysed. FDR trained as a lawyer and planned to follow his cousin Theodore into politics when the polio hit him. He was then 39 years old, and became paraplegic. He refused to let his illness limit his aims. He developed a hydrotherapy centre in Warm Springs, Georgia, which took a large slice of his fortune – in later years it became the 'winter white house'.

His willpower was so strong that he achieved his aim to succeed in politics and was elected president in 1933, 12 years after his illness struck. His example inspired thousands of polio sufferers. He used the president's annual 'Birthday Ball' to raise funds for the Warm Springs Foundation. A special Birthday Ball Commission took charge of the money. It was largely run by Paul de Kruif, whose books had already become well known. Paul was popular and highly motivated. The commission did good work with limited funds, and supported research in Harvard, Yale and John Hopkins Hospital.

However, there was not enough money so FDR initiated the first major national fund raising project in the US to create the National Foundation for Infantile Paralysis (NFIP). Its aims were to provide sufferers with the best available treatment and to raise money for research. As a national project, this was really the forerunner of the space programme. Major fundraising was undertaken – 'The March of Dimes'. Annual income reached $25million, making a total of $630million, of which 11% was set aside for research.

By the time the NFIP was winding down the main problems of polio had been solved and vaccines became available. Sadly FDR died in 1944 so he did not live to see the successful outcomes. The project was so successful a grateful congress changed the dime coin in memory of FDR by putting his image on it and releasing the coins on 30 January 30, 1946 – his birthday (Figure 4).

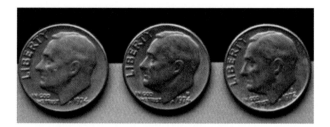

Figure 4   The March of Dimes (Newsom)

Therapy

Nothing could touch the disease, so specific therapy was concentrated on the aftermath – rehabilitation and orthopaedic surgery. Trying to maintain muscle tone and joint movements were vital. However, particularly in the 1930s resting limbs by splinting was carried to excess. The 140 nurses admitted to hospital during the Los Angeles outbreak had limbs encased in plaster by their medical colleagues anxious to do the best for them, although it turned out that few had any fever and none developed paralysis.

It would take a very vigorous personality to show that fixing limbs was wrong and graded excercises were needed, but in 1940 one appeared. Sister Kenny had been used to treating polio in the Australian outback. Her methods won great support in the US, and she soon became established as director of the Elizabeth Kenny Institute in Minneapolis. More details on her will appear in the second part of this article.

My first sight of patients with polio came in my student days with a visit to London's Western Fever Hospital. There a larger hangar had patients scattered through it encased in their 'iron lungs' (Figure 5). Paralysis had affected their breathing muscles and they required ventilation to maintain life. It was a very sobering sight.

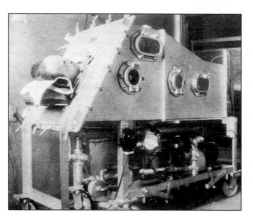

Figure 5 The 'iron lung'

The iron lung or Drinker Respirator (after Dr Philip Drinker) had been invented in Harvard in 1929. Unlike the ventilators of today, these worked by changing the pressure outside the chest, so avoiding the risks of intubation. The first was a tank, with leather seals in which the patient was nursed, and the pressure changes were provided by two vacuum cleaner motors. The noise could be heard 500 yards away. More complex machines incorporated beds and portholes, but some patients managed with a 'cuirass' ventilator, which allowed more mobility.

Interestingly in 2003 the BBC published an article on a Mr John Prestwich who had been using an iron lung for 48 years, going to St Thomas's Hospital in London for treatment. (www.johnprestwich.btinternet.co.uk)

Landmarks

In 1931 Burnet and Macnamara published a paper on the immunological differences between strains of polio virus. They showed that two 'stock' strains were different, and that when a monkey had been infected with one strain it became resistant to further infections, but remained susceptible to infection by the second strain.

Kolmer and Brodie might have had more luck with their vaccines if they had read this paper beforehand. However, it came from unknown scientists in Australia, and was given no credence in the US until the Yale team confirmed their finding.

Later a third type of virus was discovered. Sir Frank Macfarlane Burnet became a giant among scientists, and like Popper later delved into immunology developing the basic knowledge of how our immune system works. He also became a Nobel prize winner. In fact his contributions to virology and to immunology from his post at the Walter and Eliza Hall Institute in Melbourne were so numerous that his work on typing polio virus only gets one line in a 25 page biography.

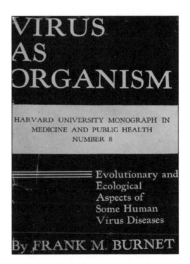

Figure 6   Burnet's lecture (1945)

Nonetheless it set the scene for typing to be used in epidemiology and vaccine production. His work on polio so impressed the Americans that in 1945 he was invited to lecture at Harvard (Figure 6), and offered a professor's post there.

The third landmark, also rewarded with the Nobel prize, was the discovery in 1949 by Enders, Weller and Robbins that polio viruses could be grown reliably in tissue culture. Enders had moved from Harvard to become director of the infectious diseases laboratory at the Boston children's hospital in 1947, and he invited the others, young men freshly out of the army, to join him.

They worked hard to develop tissue cultures for viruses, aided by the use of penicillin and later streptomycin added to the cultures to keep them bacteria-free. They used tissue from human foetuses containing skin and muscle. The test viruses were just what happened to be around at the time. The four tubes inoculated with oral washings from a case of chicken pox showed no change, but the four noculated with poliovirus showed a change in the cells that Enders called a 'cytopathic effect'. The cultures were shown to contain the virus. This meant that the way was open for research on epidemiology, immunity, and development of vaccines. When Enders was offered the Nobel prize, he refused to accept it unless his two colleagues were included 'for they did all the work', he said. Enders did not work on polio vaccines himself, but laid down the groundwork for an effective measles vaccine, for which some said he deserved a second Nobel prize.

Conclusion

Today there are worries old and new about the polio vaccine and polio itself has been the subject of great controversies. However, it is important to keep a sense of balance and remember that for many years it was a major problem. The history is well presented by one of the chief investigators from Yale, GF Paul, from whose book much of my data and the comments about Los Angeles come. The books of Paul de Kruif provide a graphic 1930s view of many aspects of infection, and are readily available online at reasonable cost. My own involvement with polio and its attendant worries continued, as will be seen in the next chapter, when development of the vaccines and the feuds/controversies surrounding them will be discussed.

Further reading

Burnet FM. Macnmara J. (1931) Immunological differences between strains of poliomyelitis virus. *Brit J Exp Path* **12**: 57–61.

de Kruif P. (1938) *The fight for life*. Jonathan Cape: London.

Enders JF. Weller TH. Robbins FC. (1949) Cultivation of the Lansing strain of poliomyelitis virus in cultures of various human embryonic tissues. *Science* **109**: 85.

Kenney E. (1941) *The treatment of Infantile Paralysis in its acute stage*. Bruce: Minneapolis.

Landsteiner K. Popper E. (1908) Mikroscopische Praparate von einem menschlichen und zwei Affenruckenmarken. *Wien klin Wschr* **21**: 1830.

Paul GF. (1971) *A History of Poliomyelitis*. Yale University Press: New Haven and London.

Chapter 18

Poliomyelitis part 2: 1950–2005 – a disease controlled (almost)

Introduction

When I reached university in 1950 polio remained a major problem, but some of the building blocks for its prevention were in place. The virus could be grown in tissue culture and so readily manipulated in the laboratory.

Monkeys (or preferably chimpanzees) were still required to test for pathogenicity and three different antigenic types of virus were known. These did not cross-protect against infection. Different strains varied in pathogenicity, an important point when selecting one for a vaccine.

Two other critical points gradually became apparent. First, the virus was present in faeces and had a faecal-oral transmission. This had been shown by the Swedes in 1911, but not accepted by the Americans until the 1940s. Finally, in 1952 virus was shown to go from the gut to the nervous system through the blood. The 'cribriform plate' much trumpeted by de Kruif finally had its come-uppance. Passage of virus through the blood could be blocked by antibodies rather than alum.

The war intervened. Polio affected armies, but the real worry was influenza (as it still is). The 'Spanish flu' epidemic of 1918–1919 involved 20 per cent of the world's population. Some 20–40 million people died including 43,000 US soldiers (more than in battle, were the Germans beaten by flu?).

In 1943 the US army understandably put resources into developing influenza vaccines, while polio took a back seat. The National Foundation for Infantile Paralysis (NFIP) still drew in funds ($8.8 million in 1945) and supported research. But O'Connor – its chief executive – asked sadly: 'What have we discovered since 1938?'

Four American scientists must be introduced: Jonas Salk, Albert Sabin, Hilary Koprowski and Thomas Francis. The first three were from immigrant families, and Francis was an 'old blood' American. Sabin (said to have become interested in microbiology after reading de Kruif's *The Microbe Hunters)* and Koprowski came from Eastern Europe. They set out to tame, or 'attenuate' wild polio viruses, and hopefully provide immunity without causing disease.

Salk – the youngest and probably the most charismatic – worked on a killed vaccine. All were supported by the NFIP, and Salk became very friendly with O'Connor – thereby ensuring continued support.

Jonas Salk

The story of Salk and his vaccine is riveting, and the subject of several books (Carter, 1967; Smith, 1990). He studied chemistry as a medical student in 1930s New York. In his final year he helped purify influenza virus in the microbiology department under Francis.

After qualification he moved to Ann Arbor in Michigan to rejoin Francis – who was setting up influenza research for the army. Salk's small salary came from the NFIP. Although he did no polio work, he learnt a lot about virology and influenza vaccine production. He was often in charge while Francis was away providing epidemiological advice for the army.

By the war's end Salk himself was advising the army. Relations with his boss became rather strained, so he moved to the Pittsburgh University Medical School, which was 'known far and wide as a dump'. He obtained enough sponsorship to found a centre of excellence where he continued his research on a killed flu vaccine. Then the NFIP sponsored a multi-centre scheme for typing isolates of polio virus. Salk saw participation as a source of funds, for a none-too-difficult job. He was soon using his influenza knowledge to start making a polio vaccine, for which he gained the support of the NFIP.

As there is no cure for polio, a vaccine was the only hope. However, it would have to be shown to be safe and effective, all at a time of intense public interest. Salk had to contend with continuous opposition from the other virologists, who thought he was a pleasant, but somewhat 'pushy' new boy, and that his concept of a killed vaccine was flawed.

His job was facilitated when the Connaught laboratories in Toronto University found a way to make concentrated virus suspensions using rhesus monkey kidney tissue cultures. They provided Salk, and later on the US drug companies, with many litres of virus suspensions.

Salk regarded inactivation of poliovirus by formalin as a chemical reaction. When performed under strictly controlled conditions (temperature/concentration of virus/acidity, etc) the virus suspension lost its viability in a semi-logarithmic fashion. The aim was to continue long enough to destroy infectivity, but leave enough virus structure to create immunity. Too long and you would get an inactive preparation, too short an infective one – so the process was critical.

By June 1952 he had three vaccines (one for each type) to test. The first few injections were given to the laboratory staff. Then he tested the vaccines in two residential homes – firstly one for those already paralysed by polio then one for the mentally retarded. The programme was carried out with amazing secrecy, although various bodies/lawyers had been involved in the 'consent' aspect (there were no research ethics committees then). The results were excellent, even those who had already had polio showed a rise in antibodies, and there were no adverse effects.

Salk continued developing his vaccines (should he include an 'adjuvant' such as mineral oil, what happened if you mixed all three types, etc), and described his results to a meeting of the NFIP virology group in January 1953. The NFIP were enthusiastic, Salk was cautiously optimistic, and the other virologists felt that many years of further research (preferably their own) was needed.

It was agreed that Salk should present his work to the scientific world in the Journal of the American Medical Association (Salk, 1953) (Figure 1), and the following week a word of caution would be published as a letter from a leading virologist saying that this was only a first step.

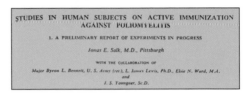

Figure 1   Salk's seminal paper

Sadly the news of a polio vaccine broke the week before the paper was published, and the NFIP bosses persuaded Salk to go on television. The medical establishment was incensed.

The NFIP then stepped into the driving seat, overruling all the virologists, Salk included – and in 1954 organised one of the largest clinical trials ever, with enthusiastic support from the 'polio pioneers' and their parents. NFIP bought vaccine from Parke Davies and Lilley (who had shown they could scale up Salk's production-protocols).

The NFIP virology advisors were largely replaced by an 'immunisation committee' who were in favour of the trial. Thomas Francis was asked to design it and given two million dollars to analyse the results. Government looked on – the only regulatory interference was an insistence that merthiolate be added to the vaccines as a preservative. Salk was furious because it made them less effective.

The trial involved some two million schoolchildren, and many more adults to look after them. Meanwhile the journalistic blitz was on. *Time* magazine had Salk on the front cover, while Paul de Kruif – now having fallen out with the NFIP – began to plant rumours that the vaccine was lethal.

However, nothing so untoward happened – the only adverse effect was allergy to the penicillin used in the tissue cultures. Francis kept the results very close to his chest. Even his staff could not predict the outcome. The polio season came and went, and at a meeting in April 1955 (on President

Roosevelt's birthday) he reported the outcome. The vaccines had been 60–80 per cent effective at preventing polio (depending on the type of virus involved). Salk was sure the relative failure was due to merthiolate, but annoyed the delegates by talking about his work on improved vaccines and not discussing the trial.

The US government was keenly interested in these results and convened a meeting of advisors in the afternoon following Francis' paper. Should the vaccine be licensed? The meeting lasted several hours, interrupted several times by phone calls from Washington asking for a decision. The answer came back – yes. However, the government took the decision to leave the polio vaccine programme in the marketplace – when they could easily have afforded to vaccinate everyone. The NFIP ordered four million doses, but then had used up all its money.

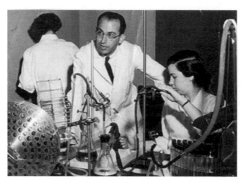

Figure 2   Jonas Salk (Carnegie Library of Pittsburgh)

Salk became a national hero. He was invited to the White House. When interviewed on national television he was asked who owned the patent. The people,' he replied, 'You might just as well try and patent the sun.'

This euphoric atmosphere was soon destroyed. Only 15 days after the vaccine was licensed some children developed polio when there was none around – 400,000 doses of vaccine had already been given. Altogether 204 people were infected, 11 of whom died. All had been vaccinated with the same batch of 'Cutter' vaccine. This company had already been in trouble for producing a batch of vaccine that had omitted one of the three types of virus. This time they had not done proper 'inactivation profiles', and indeed had already discarded several batches of vaccine because they contained living virus.

This was a major setback to the programme, an encouragement for Sabin to say 'I told you so' and continue developing a live vaccine. However, within a month four million doses of vaccine had been given with no other problems, and the programme continued to be a great success.

The UK implemented a vaccination programme with Salk vaccine made by Glaxo and Burroughs Wellcome made from less pathogenic strains of poliovirus about the time I qualified. I was vaccinated in 1958 while a trainee microbiologist in London – three injections were required. It was then that I wrote my first article on polio vaccine.

The live vaccine

Koprowski had been first in the field with a live vaccine, which was tried out in Ireland. It spread around a family (no bad thing), but worryingly polioviruses isolated from unvaccinated family members had increased pathogenicity.

In my 1958 article I commented that 'Results of trials in the Congo using this vaccine would be awaited with interest'. Koprowski had received an NFIP grant and was also supported by the Elizabeth Kenney foundation. The NFIP had given Sabin \$ 1.3 million, but had neither money nor motivation to fund another major trial, especially as the killed vaccine was working.

The live virus vaccine was therefore fostered by the World Health Organization, to whom Sabin donated his vaccine. The Sabin vaccine was tried out in Russia, and Koprowski's in Poland and the Congo – all areas where epidemics of polio occurred. The US government did not license a live virus vaccine until 1961 – and then only the Sabin strains were considered safe enough.

There were no fireworks this time, but sadly again in the US, 62 cases followed the first 21 million vaccinations; perhaps a small price to pay for the eventual eradication of polio. The live vaccine only required a sugar lump (or even just two or three drops from a vial) so was perfect for mass immunisations by unskilled volunteers.

The Far East 1958–1983

Between August 1958 and March 1959 an outbreak caused by a Type I strain of poliovirus hit Singapore, causing 415 cases. The WHO suggested a live polio vaccine. Albert Sabin had by now obtained an attenuated type II vaccine, which interfered with the ability of a type III vaccine to infect chimpanzees.

The Singapore virologists knew that the Salk vaccine would not work once an epidemic had started, and so gave the type II Sabin virus to 198,965 children. Of these only six developed polio – all but one with type I, compared with 179 out of 300,000 unvaccinated children. This was a valuable experience, because not only did the vaccine work, but it did so immediately by excluding the wild virus from the gut. Sabin wrote a long article in the *British Medical Journal* (Sabin, 1958) to allay worries that an attenuated strain might become pathogenic if passed around naturally in a community. He also noted that the Salk vaccine took time to work, failed to create immunity in infants, and probably required annual booster doses.

The summer of 1960 saw me conscripted into the army's pathology service in the Alexandra Military Hospital, Singapore. My previous training meant I was the only one who could use the laboratory Van Slyke machine that measured blood bicarbonate, a predecessor of blood gas analysis.

Everyone crowded around while I sucked some serum into a pipette (as there was no automation then). In the excitement I sucked too hard and swallowed

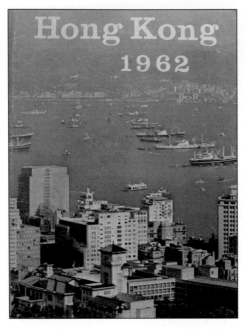

Figure 3   Hong Kong 1962 (PSI License C2009000939)

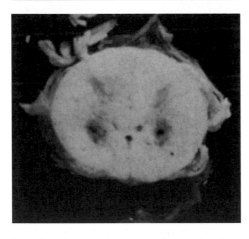

Figure 4   Autopsy specimen of a swollen spinal cord (Newsom)

some serum. The serum was from a soldier's wife with acute polio, from which she soon died (expatriates were often more at risk than local communities). Vaccination and probable previous infection notwithstanding, I spent several very anxious weeks.

Later I moved to take charge of the Army labs in Hong Kong (Figure 3). Enterovirus infection was again a problem for expatriates, and in 1962 I had the unhappy experience of performing autopsies on two British children who had died of polio. This was long before the Health and Safety at Work Act, or space travel, but I looked almost like a man on the moon. I can still remember the horrible sight of the spinal cords. The oedema meant that when they were sliced across the cut ends oozed out from the meninges and became almost mushroom shaped (Figure 4 gives an idea).

Altogether 363 cases with 52 deaths occurred in Hong Kong in 1962. A small trial of a trivalent live vaccine was performed, and showed that 96 per cent of children developed antibodies, so early in 1963 a mass vaccination programme was instituted.

I took advantage of a sugar lump, knowing that the previous killed vaccine would keep me from being one of the one in a milion infected by the oral vaccine. In a closed community such as Hong Kong at that time, even if only 50 per cent of the population received the vaccine, it would have spread to the others, and indeed no cases of polio occurred in 1963. However, not until 1983 was Hong Kong finally declared polio-free by the WHO.

Today

Today sees the 50th anniversary of the licensing of Salk's vaccine. The effect of the vaccination programme in the US is seen in Figure 5. Only 40 cases were reported in the UK between 1985 and 2000, and none since. A total of 26 of these followed vaccination with the living vaccine, and eight were in contacts of vaccines. Five were imported. An epidemic in the Caribbean country of Hispaniola in 2001, which left 28 children paralysed, was due to a vaccine strain that had reverted to being pathogenic.

Here was a catch-22 situation, because the only way to stop the outbreak was to use the live vaccine. Salk has had the last laugh, for in the UK we have returned to using a killed vaccine, which is now known to give a prolonged immunity. Interestingly enough the disease has died out in Sweden where only killed vaccine had been used, probably because of antibodies exuded into the gut from the blood of vaccinees. WHO has been pursuing an active immunisation policy using the oral vaccine, with the aid of money from Rotary International.

Surely then polio is by now consigned to history? Not so. The week I wrote this the *Financial Times* had a large photo of an indonesian baby being vaccinated

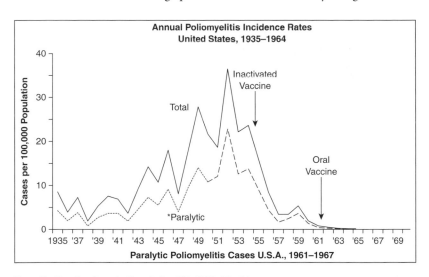

Figure 5   Results of vaccinations in the USA (CDC, Atlanta)

Thirty years of rates poliomyelitis in the United States. Data from Poliomyelitis Surveillance Reports, U.S. Public Health Service, Atlanta, Ga.

during an epidemic, the *BMJ* had seven pages on polio, and the American Society for Microbiology awarded Leslie Roberts a prize for her investigation into polio vaccination (Roberts, 2004). Also the BBC reported on the need for polio vaccine in Nigeria.

So what has gone wrong? The use of animal tissue for growing the virus always implied the possibility of contamination of the vaccines by animal viruses, hence the need for careful safety tests. Despite these, tests in 1960 revealed a 'vacuolating agent' in a batch of live virus vaccine.

This was later called SV40 (Simian Virus 40) and somewhat alarmingly was shown to cause malignant tumours when injected into hamsters. Nor was it restricted to the living vaccines – Professor Grist in Scotland found SV40 in batches of the Salk vaccine. The agent was only found in a few batches of vaccine, and excluded from future batches. There was never any evidence of tumour formation in humans, but this incident caused a lot of concern that is still being aired on the internet.

'Africans have lived with monkeys from time immemorial' is an alleged quote from Wangari Maathai, the Kenyan lady environmentalist who recently won a Nobel Prize. Why should this be relevant? Edward Hooper's theory expounded in *The River* (Hooper, 2000) (Figure 6) is that the live vaccine tested in the Congo in the 1950s, was the vehicle through which the HIV virus passed from chimpanzee to man. It is a carefully worked out plot, which traces the beginnings of Aids to the Congo, and the time when the polio vaccine was being used there. The implication is that chimpanzee tissue was used in vaccine production.

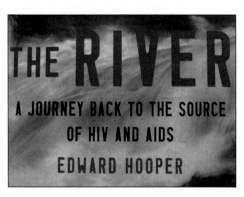

Figure 6 'The River', suggesting HIV came through polio vaccine

The book makes compelling reading. Maathai's comment relates to the alternative theory that African chimpanzee hunters were the first to be infected with Aids from chimpanzee blood.

However, Goldberg and Stricker (2005) recently suggested that the HIV-related viruses were only found in experimental chimpanzees that had been exposed to human blood. Whatever the rights and wrongs of the case – and the Centers for Disease Control, Atlanta website gives a fairly solid repudiation of it – there is no doubt that today's living vaccines do not contain HIV.

Nonetheless, some countries have viewed the oral polio vaccine with suspicion, and indeed even banned its use. In consequence of social and political opposition to the vaccine there has been a resurgence of polio in Africa and parts of India. The recent outbreak in Indonesia has been traced back to Africa via the Yemen.

Conclusion

Vaccination against polio has been a controversial topic – and remains so. The Salk/Sabin interaction has gone down as one of the great medical feuds of history. Despite the amazing outcome neither was nominated for a Nobel Prize – detractors could say that neither 'invented' their process, but adapted existing technology. Nonetheless we owe them a great deal. Even if the WHO succeeds in vaccinating everyone, for how long would vaccination be needed? What is the 'exit strategy'? The last paragraph of Paul's book written 40 years ago, starts: 'However as history is never finished, the story of poliomyelitis is not yet over.' This statement is just as true today.

Further reading

Carter R. (1967) *Breakthrough: The Saga of Jonas Salk.* Pocket Books: New York.

Goldberg B. and Stricker RB. (2005) Origin of Aids revisited. *ASM News* **71**: 157.

Hooper E. (2000) *The River.* Penguin Books: London.

Roberts L. (2004) Polio: the final assault. *Science* **303**: 1960–9.

Sabin A. (1958) The present position of immunisation against poliomyelitis with live virus vaccine. *British Medical Journal* **1**: 663–80.

Salk J. (1953) Studies in human subjects on active immunisation against poliomyelitis. *J American Medical Assn* **151**: 1081–2003.

Smith JS. (1990) *Patenting the Sun.* William Morrow: New York.

Chapter 19
Brucellosis, or Mediterranean Fever

Introduction

"Bill – your spleen has gone for a walk", said my father. I had been feverish and unwell for some time. Father sent off some of my blood, and the answer came back – 'abortus fever'. So since the age of five I've been interested in brucellosis. What is more I remember the moment of infection. My grandmother milked a friend's cow, and proudly gave me the warm milk for tea!

Brucellosis is a zoonosis – a disease of animals (mainly causing abortion) that can spread to man. Goats, cows and pigs are among those affected. The bacteria differ slightly; goats have *Brucella melitensis*, and cows have *Brucella abortus*. All this may not seem very relevant to hospital-acquired infection – but wait and see.

The name honours David Bruce, who was an army surgeon in Malta (melita – honey) at the time:

> David found a little germ
> Its name of course you know
> For everywhere that David goes
> That name is sure to go.
>
> He found it in a spleen one day
> And raised a cultured stock
> 'with you' he said 'I'll demonstrate
> the postulates of Koch'.

And so he did – transferring the disease to a monkey. David was 28, newly qualified (from Edinburgh) and newly wed, when he went to Malta. He must have been greatly helped by his wife, who was a skilled microscopist and had studied under Robert Koch in Berlin. Dr Caruana Scicluna helped with the cultures, and Bruce reported his results in 1887, calling the offending microbe *Micrococcus melitensis*.

Defining a disease

The Napoleonic wars had stimulated British interest in the Mediterranean. Malta was 'liberated' from the French in 1800, and became an increasingly important military base – especially with the Crimean war, and the opening of the Suez Canal. Fever always was a problem for the Malta garrison, which by 1904 numbered 30,000. By then fever accounted for 75,000 days of sickness per year. As early as 1869, Marston had separated 'Mediterranean gastric remittent fever' from the 'intermittent' fever of malaria, or the 'remittent' fever of typhoid. 'The accuracy of my description', he noted, 'is testified for by the patient – myself'.

Louis Hughes joined Bruce as an army doctor in 1890, remaining in Malta until 1897. That year he published the definitive description of 'Malta' fever in his monograph, calling it 'undulant fever'; a name he noted which is more acceptable to Maltese hoteliers. 'Nothing concentrates the mind' he wrote, 'like a disease one has suffered from oneself, together with wife and sister-in-law'. He dedicated the book to his friend and mentor Lord Lister. Cambridge University library has a copy datestamped 1897, but on opening it I found the pages UNCUT, and needing careful attention from a carving knife. So much for local interest in brucellosis.

Hughes' main clinical points were: an endemic, occasionally epidemic, fever with a long and indefinite duration, and undulating relapses accompanied by sweating, constipation, headache, neuralgia and swollen joints. At autopsy (mortality around 3%) the spleen was enlarged and soft (containing micrococci), but there were no gut ulcers (unlike typhoid).

Two manifestations he did not stress were endocarditis, and 'neuro-brucellosis'. One aspect of the 'cerebral' side is that with only a vague fever patients worry as to whether they really are ill – a prolonged worry can have 'psychosomatic' overtones. Florence Nightingale was never the same after her attack of 'Crimea fever', which may well have been brucellosis, and Alice Evans a famous American microbiologist who worked with brucella was labelled neurotic for 18 years before brucellosis was diagnosed.

Having defined the disease, Hughes speculated on its epidemiology. It did not seem to pass from person to person (the patient next door was safe), was not waterborne (unlike typhoid it did not attack teetotalers preferentially), nor was it related to insect bites. It did seem 'room related' so he wondered about drains, and airborne spread – concluding that it was a 'filth disease'. For treatment he recommended MILK (3.5 pints a day), as fresh and pure as possible. He noted that more people in Malta were said to drink cow's milk than there were cows. Many had goats' milk, of which he approved, supplied 'on the hoof' by the travelling goatherds; Hughes recommended Pasteurisation only if the milk could not be drunk fresh. He leaves our story to become an assistant sanitary officer in Aldershot; later he went to South Africa and was killed in action in the Boer war (aged 32).

In 1897 one more advance took place in Malta, which by then warranted an Army Professor of Pathology, Almroth Wright. He showed that brucellosis patients' serum agglutinated a suspension of brucella, and this could be used as a diagnostic test. He became Professor of Pathology at St Mary's Hospital, and a founding father of immunology – making the memorable comment: 'We must stimulate the phagocytes'.

The Mediterranean Fever Commission (MFC)

Although the disease could now be diagnosed with confidence, it occurred all around the Mediterranean and the Middle East, and there was still no idea of the cause. There were some clues – statistics from Valletta from 1897 to 1904 showed an average annual incidence per 1000 population of 36.23 for the whole garrison, 24.79 for hospital patients, and 92.4 for hospital staff. [Shades of Marston/Hughes (and a Dr Carbone who died in Italy after working on brucellosis in Malta)]. Also, officers' families were more affected.

The two main military hospitals in Malta showed a great contrast. The Army hospital in Valletta was an ancient building overlooking the Grand Harbour, taken over from the Knights of St John. Today it is a conference centre and

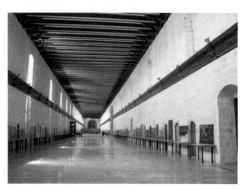

museum. The principal ward is so long it almost requires binoculars to see the end (503 feet). It is 32.5 feet high, and was regarded as an 'undesirable place to treat the sick' as it was not well ventilated. Although cool and spacious, isolating patients was impossible (Figure 1). The Naval Hospital was at Bighi, on the other side of the harbour. It was built on the cliff top in the grounds of an Italianate Villa. The hospital was built in 1830, but new

Figure 1   The Long Ward in Valetta Hospital (Newsom)

wards on the Nightingale plan were added in 1901 and 1903. Now part is in ruins, the rest the headquarters of 'Malta Heritage'. One third of the patients from the Navy were associated with Bighi.

By 1904 the UK government was concerned enough to appoint the Mediterranean Fever Commission under the auspices of the Royal Society to sort matters out. Bruce, by now a colonel and in London (editor of the *Journal of the Royal Army Medical Corps*) was made chairman; some new names from the army and navy including Horrocks (later Major-General) and Kennedy were included. Theodore Zammit was enlisted as the local bacteriologist. His laboratory has now been restored in its attic in what is now Malta's Ministry of Health. A fascinating room, it contains his desk, microscope and equipment – plus relevant letters and documents (Figure 2). A photograph on the wall shows the main members of the MFC – with Lady Bruce added (Figure 3). The Bruces spent a month back in Malta, then left for London happy that the others would be hard at work. The MFC members set to with a will – how well could the micrococcus survive – in dust, in army serge cloth, in Malta harbour water, in the sun. What about modes of infecting animals – monkeys with dust etc.?

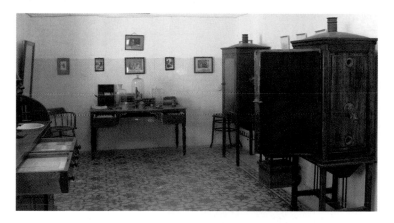

Figure 2   Zammit's laboratory – with his original desk and microscope (Newsom)

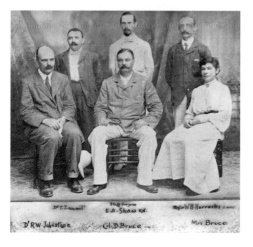

Figure 3   Some key members of the Mediterranean Fever Commission (Newsom)

Goats

Although they were well financed – the monkey supply was limited and so they looked for alternatives. Where the idea of a goat came from may never be finally known (Figure 4), but Horrocks asked Zammit to see what he could find.

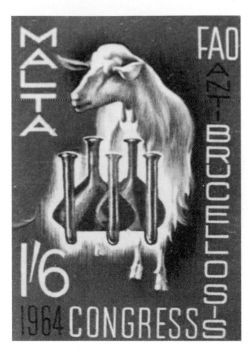

Figure 4   Maltese goals remembered

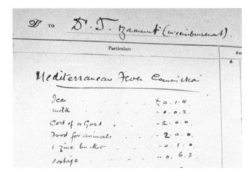

In Zammit's desk drawer is a faded MFC expenses sheet dated 20 September 1904, including 'Goat £2.0.0.' (Figure 5). His first experiment was to test the blood of this 'white goat' for brucella agglutinins. The result was negative, and so on 18 September he fed the goat with a brucella culture. Six weeks later the goat's blood contained agglutinins. He repeated this in December on a 'red goat', again with no agglutinins beforehand, but these appeared two weeks later. By April 1905 the white goat was still well, and he wrote: 'These two experiments led me to the belief that goats are susceptible to Malta fever, and the disease may be spread to human beings by goats' (Figure 6). So in June 1905 he examined the blood of six goats from two herds – five reacted strongly with the brucella cultures.

Re-enter Horrocks – he re-tested the bloods and confirmed Zammit's observations. He was able to buy the animals cheaply as they 'had given very little milk for some time'. He examined the five positive goats, and found abundant micrococci in the milk, but none in the urine. He then asked Captain Kennedy to check blood (with the owner's consent) from different herds in the island – 84 out of 161 goats tested gave a reaction. Horrocks himself then tested some of the herds that assembled outside hospital gates every morning. He found plenty of evidence of brucellas in the milk.

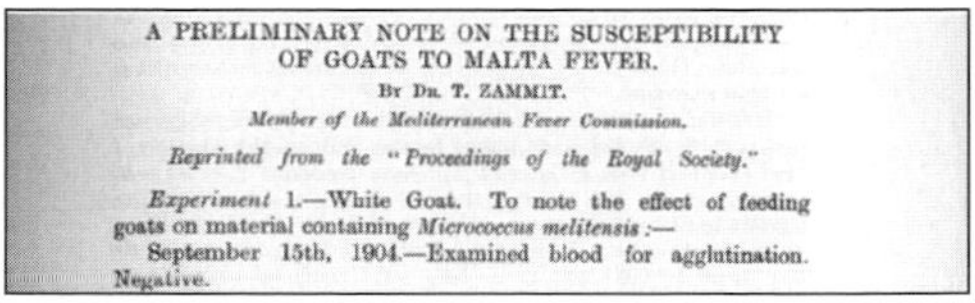

A PRELIMINARY NOTE ON THE SUSCEPTIBILITY OF GOATS TO MALTA FEVER.
By Dr. T. ZAMMIT.
Member of the Mediterranean Fever Commission.
Reprinted from the "Proceedings of the Royal Society."
Experiment 1.—White Goat. To note the effect of feeding goats on material containing *Micrococcus melitensis* :—
September 15th, 1904.—Examined blood for agglutination. Negative.

Figure 6   Zammit's original paper – 230 words long

The goat theory was supported by two independent observations. Horrocks noted that 'Rock' fever, which affected the Gibraltar garrison, disappeared in 1904 after Maltese goats (imported and used for years for milk) had been replaced by local goats due to increased shipping and grazing costs (Figure 7). The fame of the Maltese goats had reached the USA, whose government sent an agricultural officer, Mr Thompson, in 1905 to purchase a herd, as the foundation of an American industry. Sixty-five goats were shipped on the SS *Joshua Nicholson*. By the time it reached Amsterdam eight of the 12 crew on board had acquired brucellosis (the others either boiled the milk or didn't drink it). On arrival in New Jersey the goats were quarantined. One American woman who drank the milk in the quarantine station became infected, and poor Mr Thompson died. The remaining goats were slaughtered.

In June 1906 the Commission members began a 'ban goats' milk', campaign. As might be expected this ran into fierce opposition from both users and suppliers. Even other army doctors were sceptical. Ross, from the Sanitary Department of Port Said, did his own investigation in Malta and decided that brucellosis must be insect borne. He noted that sailors only contracted the disease on-shore and: 'The British Sailor does not as a rule, when he goes on shore at night on the spree, drink MILK.' Nonetheless a complete ban for the military came into force in Malta in July 1906, and the results were stunning (Figure 8). Zammit built on his success by becoming a famous archaeologist, and later rector of the university, and became Sir Theodore. Bruce continued a career in military tropical medicine, and discovered the cause of sleeping sickness – *Trypanosoma brucei*; and finally became the Surgeon-General of the British Army.

The Maltese were less impressed – Kennedy reprinted comments from the local papers. One telling one: 'Why do these bacteriologists not go back to their homes and suggest to their consumptive countrymen not to drink the milk of cows, which contains the bacillus of Koch'. Or 'Why instead of inventing Maltese fevers do they not suggest to their countrymen not to overtire themselves under the scorching rays of the sun playing the savage game called Rugby, and immediately after dipping into ice-cold water, or drinking whiskey that would burn even a stomach made of marble'; 'They should not recommend us to boil the milk, which while destroying the germs in the milk destroys the better qualities our milk has that has invigorated our forefathers and our children'.

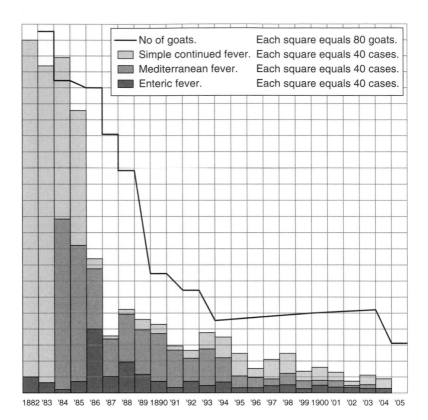

Figure 7 Horrocks' Gibraltar statistics showing the decline of Malta fever

Year	Civil		Navy		Army	
	Cases	Deaths	Cases	Deaths	Cases	Deaths
1901 642		51	252	3	253	9
1902 624		45	354	2	155	6
1903 589		48	339	6	404	9
1904 573		50	333	8	320	12
1905 663		88	270	7	643	10
1906 822		117	145	4	163	2
1907 714		78	12	0	9	1
	4,627	489	1,705	30	1,947	55

Table 1 Cases of Brucellusis and Deaths among the Civilian and Military Population of Malta during the period 1901–1907 (Eyre)

Figure 8 Results of the ban on milk in 1906

Brucellosis – worldwide

Cows worldwide were also known to have contagious abortion, and in 1897 Dr Bang isolated a bacillus from the cow's placenta. As well as its shape, it differed from Bruce's micrococcus as it required carbon dioxide for growth. Kennedy, back in London in 1914, found agglutinins for *Micrococcus melitensis* in cows, but the first war supervened. The scene moved to the USA, where Alice Evans finally showed that Bang's bacillus, and Bruce's micrococcus were related, and called them both 'Brucella' (in 1918) deciding that both were actually 'bacilli'. Even then it was another ten years before 'undulant fever' in humans was attributed to cows' milk (in Rhodesia). *Brucella suis* was also found in the USA from pigs. As we saw with tuberculosis – pasteurisation of milk was slow to take off, and while a vaccine (S19) for cows became available, one for goats was more problematic.

Makdour in his 1990 review of brucellosis noted that only 17 countries in the world (including the Channel Islands), were free of brucellosis by 1985. Even after introduction of pasteurisation, raw milk (from both cows and goats) has been used for cheese making as it is still today. Brucellosis has now been eradicated in Malta – the last major epidemics related to goats' cheese. Nearer home – a patient in St Thomas's Hospital developed brucellosis while recovering from open-heart surgery. His Italian family had sent him a goats-milk cheese to cheer him up.

Occupational exposure

Laboratory technicians

Three infections occurred in 1897 in a UK Army laboratory, to which Hughes had sent cultures, and by 1907 a further eight infections were reported. Three were needlestick injuries, two from use of a pipette, and two were deliberate self-inoculation (dislike of army life? suicide?). By far the largest laboratory outbreak showed a potential for airborne spread. It occurred (in 1938) in a university building in Michigan with a brucella research wing in the basement. There were 45 clinical cases (one death) and 49 subclinical infections. Nearly all were students, although a 'rep' who just called in with some literature on two occasions, was also infected. There was an unprotected centrifuge at the foot of the stairwell, used to process brucella cultures, and it seems likely that some massive aerosols were generated by it.

Veterinary, farm, and abattoir workers

These have all been at risk, both from contact, and from aerosols generated by handling infected animals. My own knowledge of vets suggests they have a high index of suspicion, and become very worried.

Conclusion

Brucellosis has been vanquished from much of the world, but prevalence in many countries is still unknown. I diagnosed brucellosis in an Arabian potentate who had been referred to the haematologists in Cambridge with a large spleen, and it is certainly still widespread in east Africa.

An internet search on abebooks.com reveals another worrying aspect. For sale: Speech of Major-General Abdul Karim Qassim – chief of Iraq's armed forces – who was killed in 1963, executed by orders of Saddam Hussein, possibly already ill as an alleged target of the CIA – allegedly sent a presentation handkerchief, laced with brucellosis. Probably fantasy land, but sadly brucella is now on the list of bioterrorist germs.

Father managed to obtain some M&B 693 (sulphanilamide) for me, the first of the new sulphonamides. It worked, although I now realise there was only a 30% chance of success. More effective antibiotic therapy is now available, but it is to be hoped that the rest of the world will follow the Maltese example in disease eradication.

Acknowledgement

I am grateful to Dr Michael Borg, Consultant in Hospital Infection Control, St Luke's Hospital, Malta, and Chairman of the International Federation of Infection Control, for information and showing me round the sites in Malta.

Further reading

Hughes ML. (1897) *Mediterranean, Malta, or undulant fever.* Macmillan: London.
Kennedy JC. (1907) A little humour from the Malta Fever Commission. *Journal of the Royal Army Medical Corps* **9**: 594–8.
Makdour MM. (1989) *Brucellosis.* Butterworths: London.
Mediterranean Fever Commission. Reports of the Commission appointed by the Admiralty, the War Office, and the civil government of Malta, for the investigation of Mediterranean Fever, under the supervision of an advisory committee of the Royal Society. Harrison: London, 1905 (reprinted in the *Journal of the Royal Army Medical Corps* 1904–1907).

Chapter 20

Tuberculosis part 1: defining a disease and its social consequences

Introduction

Tuberculosis (TB) is a very ancient disease. Although it was not documented in pictures as well as the 'club foot' of polio, we have hard evidence of the disease in Mummies from both Egypt and Peru, and other old human bones. Somehow the infection must have crossed the land bridge between Alaska and Europe before the continents parted.

Unlike polio, TB is widespread throughout the animal kingdom, and fossils record lesions in animals from prehistoric times. However, animals tend to have their own strains of tubercle bacilli.

Humans today are mainly affected by the human strain of *Mycobacterium tuberculosis* and spread is from human to human, but in the past bovine TB was common due to drinking infected cows milk.

The distribution today is paradoxical. In my last year as a chest hospital microbiologist, I only saw ten cases of TB, and my successor saw none in the first six months of 2006.

Indeed, from 2000 to 2003 only 0.04% of NHS bed days were devoted to tuberculous patients. Nonetheless the World Health Organization declared a global emergency in 1993 when one-third of the world's population was estimated to be infected. In 2004, deaths (especially in Africa) reached around two million – more than those from acquired immune deficiency syndrome (Aids) and nine million new cases were reported.

The arrival of multi-drug-resistant (MDR) strains in New York, with infectivity for healthcare workers created a sensation similar to that from severe acute respiratory syndrome (SARS). MDR precautions (ventilated rooms/respirators etc.) outdid those for methicillin-resistant *Staphylococcus aureus* (MRSA), and indeed in one US hospital the incidence of staphylococcal infection as measured by numbers of bacteraemias rose once MDR precautions were implemented using facilities previously dedicated to nursing MRSA patients.

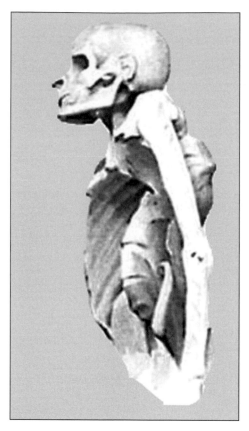

Figure 1   An Egyptian Mummy with spinal tuberculosis (Newsom)

Mycobacterium means 'fungus-like bacterium' and mycobacteria are related to actinomycetes, which are true fungi. *Mycobacterium tuberculosis* is unusual in that it has a thick and fatty cell wall, and probably because of this it takes a long time to grow and is hard to stain.

These properties are reflected in the disease. The normal body defence cells sweep up invading bacteria in the primary infection, but instead of destroying them and forming pus – they protect them and the bacteria survive happily – usually in the lungs, often to cause recurrent disease. The slow multiplication makes for a chronic disease, but usually allows the body time to wall off the infection.

The outcome of infection depends on a complex interaction between the bacteria and the body defences. The study of this interaction formed the starting place for cellular immunology. The classical picture was of a grandfather sitting by the fireside spitting over the baby on the rug. Both would soon die, as neither had much immunity.

Often the 'primary' infection seems to be no more than 'flu'. As a medical student in pre-BCG days, I turned out to be 'mantoux-positive', although I had had no significant illness. A total of 50% of my group were also positive – so at that time seemingly half the UK population must have been infected. We were nonetheless a healthy group.

So far so good, but we have the awful example of Eleanor Roosevelt (wife of the US president), who died from TB. In her case she was infected in her youth, but lived a healthy life. However, when aged 74 she was given steroids for aplastic anaemia, her immune state was compromised, and she died from the disease. The bacteria must have survived within her for many years.

Naming the infection

In contrast to the 'Black Death', Dubos' description of the 'White Plague' suggests pallor, youth and innocence. John Keats, who died aged 26 in 1821, wrote: 'Youth grows pale and spectre thin, and dies.' John Bunyan called consumption 'The Captain of all these men of death'.

However, the earliest description of pulmonary TB was probably that of 'consumption', originally found in Hindu writings of 1500BC to 2000BC. The Bible records Moses warning the children of Israel that if they transgressed: 'The Lord will smite you with consumption and with fever...' Hippocrates recognised 'consumption', and made the connection with bone disease. He wrote: 'It occurs between the ages of 18 and 35' – suggesting a widespread prevalence. He called the growths in the lungs 'tubercula' because they looked like small potatoes, and may also have coined the term 'pthisis', which was used for many centuries afterwards.

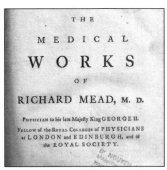

Figure 2   Richard Mead's works – dated 1767 (Newsom)

Galen, the Greek physician who lived in Rome thought that consumption was contagious, although he discounted airborne spread in favour of 'fomites'. Around AD170, he described a commonsense therapy of diet, fresh air, sea voyages, and dry elevated places. Little changed during the many centuries of the 'dark ages'.

Another obvious manifestation of TB was 'scrofula'; infection of lymph nodes (from bovine TB bacteria), usually appearing as painless lumps in the neck (Latin: scrofa = brood sow). It could progress to ulceration and produce terrible scars.

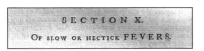

Figure 3   Hectick Fever – from Richard Mead (Newsom)

The 'divine right' of Kings fostered the custom of 'touching' to cure disease. Scrofula was pre-eminent among diseases to be cured by touch, and became called the 'King's Evil'. King Clovis included 'touching' at his coronation in AD496, but it did not become common in England until the reign of Edward the Confessor in the 11th century.

Some 600 years later the practice still persisted – King Charles II was said to have 'touched' 92,102 subjects, and Queen Anne – the last monarch to continue this tradition included the famous Dr Johnson (as a child) among her patients.

The 'divine right' did not extend to the King's own health – Edward VI had scrofula and probably died of TB in 1553 after a reign of only six years.

Several advances were made in the 1700s. Richard Morton, a London physician, used the term 'tuberculosis' implying the lesions were 'tubercles', and the term 'miliary tuberculosis' was used to describe the widespread lesions that sometimes follow primary infection complicated by septicaemia, which were the size of 'millet seeds'.

The cheesy dead material found in old lung abscesses was called 'caseous', and its production became 'caseation'. My copy of the 1767 edition of the works of Richard Mead (famous for his views on smallpox) devotes three pages to the 'slow or hectick fevers' of consumption. He recommends 'asses milk' as being 'more cooling and detergent', and notes that patients with lung infection 'are very justly sent to Lisbon or Naples'. If this is not possible, he suggests 'riding on horseback'.

The social impact of tuberculosis

When childhood infection was common, some died early, but most (like myself) suppressed the infection. Adolescence produced a further stress, when dormant microbes could gain the upper hand or be reinforced by secondary infections. Before therapy, many, like Edward VI, would die young.

World-ranking artists whose careers were cut short by illness illustrate the seriousness of the disease. The cover from Dormandy's excellent book shows some of the Bronte sisters – all five Bronte children died by the age of 37.

The well-documented life of Keats illustrates the ravage of the disease. His mother died of tuberculosis when he was 14 years old. Later he studied medicine, and although he qualified, he was much more interested in poetry – one of his best poems was written during a pathology lecture (on the hob-nailed liver).

The year he qualified (1818) he nursed his younger brother who died from TB in his arms. The following year, he wrote nearly all his best poetry, but in February 1820 he returned home one evening looking so ill that his roommate sent him straight to bed. The latter recalled: 'Before his head touched the pillow, he coughed and I heard him say: '"This is blood"... "Bring me a candle Brown, and let me see this blood"'. He examined the blood and looked up with a calmness of countenance I can never forget and said: "This is arterial blood, I cannot be deceived by its colour, it is my death warrant".

Therapy at that time consisted of venesection to remove blood, and a starvation diet – both of which must have reduced his resistance to infection. Fortunately he was seen by a noted physician, Robert Bree, in March. Bree, who owned one of the few stethscopes in the UK, said he had been misdiagnosed and should get up, take exercise and have a good diet.

This gave Keats several happy and productive months respite. Was this a misdiagnosis? One suggestion is that Bree was a humane man, who could see that the disease was likely to be fatal, and saw no need for such enervating treatment.

However, by September, haemorrhages had returned and the thought of another winter in England was daunting.

His friend and contemporary poet Percy Bysse Shelley (who also suffered from TB) invited him to Rome. Shelley wrote: 'Consumption is a disease particularly fond of people who write such good verse as you have done, and with the assistance of the English winter it can often indulge the selection. I do not think young and amiable poets are at all bound to gratify its taste; they have entered into no bond with the muses to that effect.'

Rome was said to have a good English doctor – Sir James Clarke (who became physician to Queen Victoria). So with a heavy heart, Keats said farewell to his fiancée and in September set off by boat for Rome accompanied by Joseph Severn, a young painter.

The voyage was horrendous – it took ten days to get to Portsmouth. They finally arrived at Naples a month later, where Keats had to stay on board for a ten-day quarantine.

Clarke found them lodgings at the foot of the Spanish steps, and did his best to encourage Keats, but the latter was by now

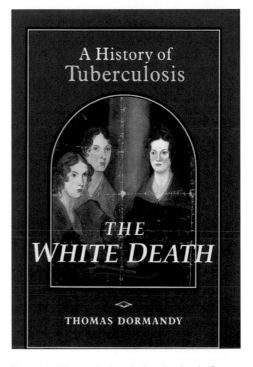

Figure 4   A history of tuberculosis – showing the Bronte sisters (by Thomas Dormandy)

having repeated haemorrhages, and spent much of his time in bed. He died on 21 February 1821. 'He called out: "Severn lift me up for I am dying. I shall die easy... do not be frightened."'

Severn's letters paint a horrendous picture. 'Our landlady has called the police, to say he has consumption. If he dies all his belongings will be burnt.' 'The money is running out – we only have £70 left' (Clarke paid the rent).

Severn made a haunting sketch of the dying poet, but he himself lived on in Rome for many years, becoming a successful painter. Shelley died in a boating accident not long after Keats, and all three are buried in nearby plots in the Testaccio cemetery (Cimitero Protestante) in Rome.

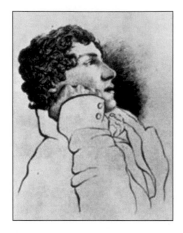

Figure 5   John Keats in 1819 (sketch by Charles Brown)

The house at the foot of the Spanish steps was bought in 1903 by the Keats-Shelley Memorial Association and has become a museum well worth visiting (Keats's bed was not burnt and remains there). The top floors of the house are run by the 'Landmark' trust, and can be booked for short stays in Rome.

Similar stories could be told about many artists – Chopin, for instance, was turned out of Majorca when his 'consumption' was recognised. Aubrey Beardsley died on the French Riviera in 1898, aged 25 after an amazingly productive life – finally repentant about his more erotic sketches.

But not all ended in disaster. Robert Louis Stevenson was treated by another Dr Clarke – he was recommended to leave Edinburgh for warmer climates, and like many others spent the winter on the French Riviera. He recovered enough to return and become a barrister. However, his disease fluctuated. He had many visits to the Riviera, and spent some years in Davos in Switzerland, which had become a major centre for treating TB.

Later he had a relapse and was sent to Colorado. He finally ended up in Tahiti, where his sudden death was probably due to a cerebral haemorrhage unrelated to his TB.

He wrote: 'I have a little shadow that goes in and out with me, And what can be the use of him is more than I can see.'

Authors and musicians from Shakespeare onwards have included tragic figures in their writings. In La Boheme, Mimi's story was taken from the life of a poor Parisian flower girl, who became a friend of the author.

Sanatoria inspired several books; the most famous, *The Magic Mountain* by Thomas Mann describes life (and death) in Davos, where his wife was treated for

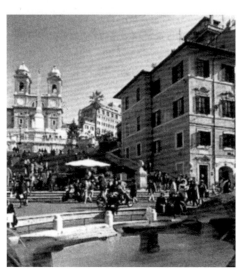

Figure 6   Rome – the Spanish Steps and the Keats–Shelley Museum (Newsom)

TB. It is a long interesting book, with a tense – 'will our hero survive?' aspect. At the end is a stern message from author to reader: 'You read this book for the story, but I wrote it for the philosophy – so now you know the story – read the book again.'

Defining the disease

Auenbrugger
In the 18th century, the industrial revolution concentrated people in cities and increased the incidence of TB. The 'renaissance' replaced the 'dark ages' and the time was ripe for advances in 'phthisisology'.

Leopold von Auenbrugger was the son of an innkeeper in Graz (Austria) whose wife was very musical.

Auenbrugger noted that his father could tell how much wine was left in a barrel by tapping it. When he became a doctor, he applied the same principle to the chest. This must have been a major breakthrough at a time when medicine relied on symptoms, and physical examination was eschewed. Like his mother he was musical, and indeed wrote a successful opera for which he was ennobled and invited to court in Vienna. His talent enabled him to use 'percussion' to define consolidation in the chest, and delineate cavities.

In 1761 he wrote 'Inventum Novum', which however might have vanished for all time, but for the French professor Corvisart who read of it 30 years later. One of Corvisart's students was Renée Laennec (1781–1826).

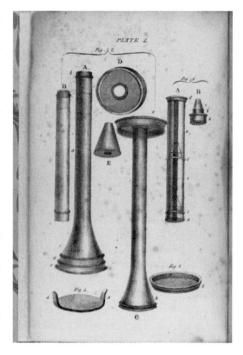

Figure 7   Laennec's plans for a stethoscope (Wellcome Images)

Laennec
Nothing stimulates study of a disease like suffering from it oneself. Laennec died of TB, but not before he had made a major contribution to medicine – the stethoscope. A qualified doctor, he came to Paris in 1801, where he led a full life despite poverty and illness: 'In his poor lodgings he would sit writing at his desk, naked to the waist to overcome his profuse sweating.'

He wrote a thesis on the writings of Hippocrates, studied in the autopsy room, taught students, edited medical journals, engaged in lively controversies, and contributed original papers to the literature. His major contribution to the pathology of TB came from the autopsy room.

By careful observations from over 200 autopsies, he described all the different manifestations of the pulmonary disease – infiltrates, tubercles and cavities – all within three years of his arrival in Paris. He found tubercles in other parts of the body too, and in 1839 Professor Schoenleim in Zurich reiterated Morton and suggested that the disease should be called 'tuberculosis' rather than phthisis.

By 1818 Laennec was a well-established Paris consultant. While he knew that direct auscultation of the chest was possible, decorum prevented him from applying it – especially to a fat young female such as his patient Mlle de Surenne, in whom percussion was useless.

A visit to the gardens of the Louvre stimulated his already prepared mind. He saw some boys playing a game remembered from childhood. Two groups were playing at opposite ends of a log. One would scratch an end with a pin, and the others would laugh when they heard the noise at the other end: 'I therefore took a paper notebook, rolled it up tightly, applied one end to the precardiac region and listened at the other. I was as surprised as I was pleased to hear the heart beat much more clearly and distinctly.'

By 1819 he had developed a more substantial instrument using a lathe, and was able to describe the different sounds he had heard and relate them to diseases in the heart and chest. Often he used postmortem findings to substantiate his diagnoses. His fame spread and in 1822 he became Regius Professor, but

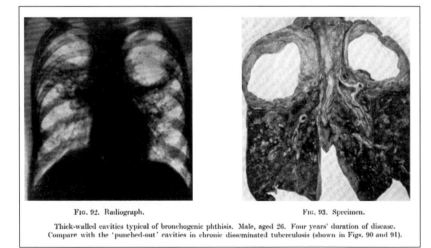

FIG. 92. Radiograph.   FIG. 93. Specimen.

Thick-walled cavities typical of bronchogenic phthisis. Male, aged 26. Four years' duration of disease. Compare with the 'punched-out' cavities in chronic disseminated tuberculosis (shown in Figs. 90 and 91).

Figure 8   Chest x–ray showing large apical cavities in the lungs, and then the autopsy specimen of the lungs from a young man who died like Keats in his 26th year

disease lurked in the wings – three years later, his tuberculosis produced cavities. He left Paris for his country home, but only survived until August 1826.

Roentgen
Wilhelm Conrad Roentgen was Professor of Physics in Wurzburg University. On 8 November 1895, he was experimenting on the passage of an electric current through a vacuum tube. The tube was enveloped in black cardboard.

To his surprise, he saw some crystals on a nearby bench fluoresce. He put a book, some timber, and some glass between the tube and the crystals, which still fluoresced. Finally he put his hand in the way and became the first human to see living bones outlined.

This discovery was soon developed. Within a year, Thomas Edison had produced the X–ray fluoroscope. Now tuberculous lesions of the lungs could be visualised – sometimes before the patient had any symptoms.

A major outcome from this was use of mass-miniature X-ray to screen whole populations for the disease. Roentgen was a modest man, who did not patent his invention. However, he was eventually rewarded by the Nobel Prize, some four years before Robert Koch.

Conclusion
Tuberculosis has probably had more effect on mankind than any other illness. With this in mind it is impossible in this article to do more than sketch out the major topics and developments throughout history.

Part two will consider the search for a cause, the epidemiology with special reference to healthcare workers, prevention and cure.

Further reading

Further reading on history:

Daniel T. (1977) *Captain of death: the story of tuberculosis.* University of Rochester Press: Rochester.
Dormandy T. (1999) The white death. The Hambledon Press: London.
Dubos R. Dubos J. (1953) The white plague. Victor Gollancz, London.

Further reading on sanatorium life in the 1900s:

Mann T. (1928) *The magic mountain (Der Zauerberg).* Secker M. (transl.) (1985) Penguin Books: Harmondsworth.

Chapter 21
Tuberculosis part 2: finding the cause and trying to eliminate it

Introduction

The plot thickens. I have already mentioned multiple-drug-resistant (MDR) strains of *Mycobacterium tuberculosis*. The drastic control measures taken in the US were followed by a reduction in cases, and are recommended in the National Institute for Health and Clinical Excellence (NICE) guidelines on tuberculosis published by the Royal College of Physicians (2006).

Nevertheless, we now have extensively drug resistant (XDR) strains, which are also resistant to some of the 'third line' drugs used to treat MDR infections. Of 17,690 isolates from reference laboratories throughout the world in 2000 to 2005, 20% were MDR and 2% were XDR.

XDR strains were found as far apart as the US, South Korea and Latvia (Morbidity and Mortality Weekly Report, 2006). The potential danger of XDR strains is shown in an outbreak in South Africa, 52 of 53 patients (all with HIV) died within a median of 25 days. All had been in hospital previously, raising the likelihood of nosocomial infection – this was a real 'wake-up call' (Lawn and Wilkinson, 2006).

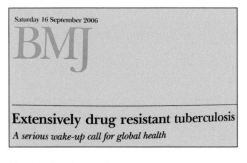

Saturday 16 September 2006

BMJ

Extensively drug resistant tuberculosis
A serious wake-up call for global health

Figure 1   A wake-up call

However, back to history. Was the disease familial or contagious? Hippocrates mentioned the phthisic diathesis. The occurrence of the disease in families (the Keats' for example) and the high death rate in small children (grandfather coughing over the baby) suggested a genetic element.

Galen thought phthisis was contagious and later Benjamin Marten (1722) wrote in *A new theory of consumptions*: 'The original and essential cause may possibly be certain species of animalculi or wonderfully minute living creatures that by their peculiar shape or disagreeable parts are inimical to our nature… Worms and animalculi fretting and gnawing.'

The search for a cause

The situation was complicated by infections caused by human (generalised or pulmonary tuberculosis) and bovine (lupus or gut tuberculosis) tubercle bacilli. These also differ in cultural characteristics and their effects on animals (bovine is bad for bunnies!). Thus it is not surprising that errors occurred en route.

Although Laennec doubted the 'contagious' theory, another Frenchman, Antoine Villemin was one of the first to prove it. He was an army doctor, who being in the cavalry recognised that glanders (in horses) was definitely contagious. He thought that tuberculosis, which was common among the soldiers, resembled glanders, and so in 1865 he successfully infected rabbits from humans, and showed that material from an infected cow gave a more serious infection in the rabbit. His views were largely ignored.

Edwin Klebs ('klebsiella') confirmed Villemin's findings by transferring the 'monas tuberculosum' to an animal, but definitive proof had to wait until Robert Koch's work. By 1881 Koch was well prepared. He was in Berlin, well-funded by the government with his 'state of the art' technology – the microscope fitted with a condenser and an oil-immersion lens. He could see stained bacteria and make cultures. Nonetheless the speed with which he worked was amazing, the more so because of the slow growth and stain-resistance of tubercle bacilli. He started work on 18 August 1881 and was delivering his 'famous and historic lecture' to the Berlin Physiological Society on 24 March 1882.

By then he had demonstrated bacteria in human tissue (he had to stain for 24 hours using dye and caustic potash), grown them on coagulated beef serum, and reproduced the disease by injecting human material and cultures into animals. He had set up 43 cultures and infected 79 guinea pigs, 35 rabbits, and four cats.

The news travelled fast – a copy of the weekly *Berlin Medical Journal* appeared on John Tyndall's desk in London on 10 April. He summarised Koch's results in a letter to *The Times*, which was printed on 22 April and re-printed by the *New York Times* two days later. The news warranted accompanying editorials in both papers. Only in France did it take another six months to surface in a newspaper – *L'Echo*.

Paul Ehrlich was so stimulated by Koch's lecture that the same evening he began the researches on staining that eventually led to the 'Zeihl Neelson' technique, whereby a very strong red stain was used. The material surrounding the bacilli was then decolourised with acid and then alcohol, and counterstained.

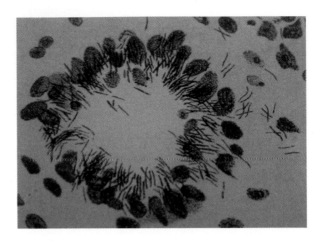

Figure 2   Koch's original preparation showing tubercle bacilli stained blue (Newsom)

Today fluorescent techniques are used, but the decolourising stage remains, and one way to refer to tuberculosis (TB) (especially when you do not want patients to know) is to talk of acid-fast disease.

Later Koch's cholera studies took him to India, where he continued his work on TB. He noted the lethal effect of sunlight (UV) on tubercle bacilli, but also recorded that they could survive for 43 days in putrefying sputum and 186 days in dried sputum. He performed many more cultures and animal experiments, importantly showing that inhalation was a significant route of infection.

He published a definitive paper in 1884, which was translated into English and appears together with his other work in *Microparasites and disease* (Koch, 1886). He concluded that therapy was 'not in prospect', and so we should concentrate on prophylaxis – by disinfection, and by 'preservation of healthy persons from contact with the bacilli'.

Bovine tuberculosis I

Koch had grown the bovine tubercle bacilli, and confirmed Villemin's finding that they differed from human strains. Villemin reported transmission of bovine TB to humans at the first international TB Congress in Paris in 1888. By then pasteurisation of milk had begun, and delegates recommended it together with slaughter of obviously diseased animals. This would have stopped bovine infection in humans completely.

However, at the second international Congress in 1901, Koch produced a 'bolt from the blue' by stating that human TB did not affect cows, and it was unlikely that bovine TB affected humans. Lord Lister, who was in the chair, was astonished. Here was the world authority making a dogmatic statement.

Lister made some off-the-cuff comments, concluding that: 'The congress would probably require a more searching inquiry...,' and followed this up with a letter to the *British Medical Journal* ending with 'that bovine TB is not communicable to man, there is I venture to think no reliable evidence'.

Koch's announcement completely paralysed all public health projects to stamp out bovine TB. A Royal Commission was set up to study the problem in the UK. The members included German Sims Woodhead (founder of Papworth Village Settlement and professor of Pathology at Cambridge). They were well funded and facilities included an experimental farm. After ten years work they reported that bovine TB did in fact affect humans. An unexpected spin-off was the establishment of the Medical Research Council (MRC).

Tuberculin

In 1889 Koch disappeared into his laboratory and shut the door. Then he announced that he had obtained a substance he called tuberculin, which he implied was a cure for tuberculosis. The great Koch had a cure. Trains from the French Riviera were booked out for months ahead as thousands of sufferers flocked to Berlin. Lister brought his niece for treatment.

Conan Doyle (a doctor as well as the originator of Sherlock Holmes) went to investigate. He found a pile of letters on the floor, as high as a man's knee and four feet across, which he was told represented a single post. He was sceptical and thought the 'cure' might be better as a diagnostic agent.

Koch never claimed that tuberculin killed the bacteria, but said that it created an inflammation around the diseased tissue and allowed the normal body defences access to the bacilli. Undoubtedly he was correct in saying that tuberculin created an inflammation. Unfortunately in many cases this allowed the bacteria to break out and overcome the body defences, so worsening the illness.

It was out of character for Koch to have produced a 'secret' cure (it turned out to be a filtrate of a culture of tubercle bacilli, suspended in glycerine and evaporated to 1/50th of its volume), and to have announced it prematurely.

The suggestion is that his employers (the government) had pressurised him. Possibly his domestic situation (divorce/remarriage to a student) made his attention wander. He certainly did not do it for the money – there is no evidence he made any at all from it.

Conan Doyle turned out to be correct. As immunity to tuberculosis turned out to be cell mediated, no blood tests were available, and the 'tuberculin test' (first used in 1905, now the Mantoux test) became the basic diagnostic test for tuberculosis – especially where bacteria could not be seen or grown.

Bovine tuberculosis II

As by 1907 both tuberculin testing for cows and pasteurisation of milk had become established, eradication of bovine TB was possible. However, in the UK there was not enough money for a 'test and slaughter' programme, and many people objected to the taste of pasteurised milk. 'A few germs do you good' was the message.

Even in 1923 around 10% of deaths from TB in the UK and 33% of those in the under-fives were due to the bovine type. A total of 2,500 died in 1934, when 40% of dairy cows were still infected. It was not surprising that US soldiers in the 1940s were forbidden to drink English milk.

Gradually a campaign got under way so that by 1960 nearly all herds were accredited. Even today up to 3% of milk is not pasteurised (especially that used for some tasty cheese). Only nine isolates of bovine bacilli were made in 2002 from humans in the UK (and may well have been from immigrants).

Tuberculin testing of cattle is ongoing, but in 2002 19,792 cows tested positive. Why? One suggestion is that they become infected from badgers. Badger culling

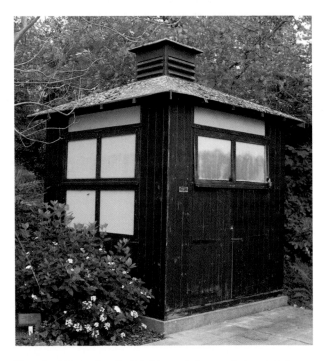

Figure 3   A Papworth patient's hut (one set of upper windows had always to be open) (Newsom)

has been tried, and is an emotive subject. Other animals such as deer might also be involved (as are possums in New Zealand). A recent (2009) report from Northern Ireland revealed that bovine TB in cows has *increased* since 1997, and regarded eradication as a long-term goal.

A small outbreak of bovine TB in children occurred in an Oxfordshire village some years ago. Investigation revealed they drank raw milk. Although the herd concerned had been accredited, re-testing showed that many had converted. How had the cows become infected? It turned out that the herdsman had had bovine TB many years earlier.

Therapy

Although many recovered naturally (like me) from a primary infection, 50% of those with active TB died within two years. Fresh air, rest and building resistance (a pint of milk a day!) were the mainstays of treatment, and generated the 'sanatorium' movement. Papworth was unique in providing therapy, accommodation and work in one village setting, and thanks to the vision of its founder, Pendrill Varrier Jones (the Pendragon) it succeeded.

Those who might well have remained at work hiding their illness in order to provide for their families (a danger to fellow workers) were housed and treated in a self-help community. Many of the houses in the village were built by patients. Even in the 1960s the hospital had a 'family' atmosphere, as although it was an NHS hospital many of the staff were original patients or members of their families had been.

Seeing half of those around you dying despite medical care must have been very disheartening – so why not try 'Steven's Cure' (Newsom, 2002) or 'Umckaloabo'. As a tuberculous 17 year old in Birmingham, Stevens had been told: 'You are for it my lad, unless you go to the veldt in South Africa.' There he met the witch doctor who gave him the infusion (of a pelargonium root). He returned healthy to Wimbledon and set up shop. His main advert was 'a cure, or your money back'.

In 1908 he suggested to the Brompton Hospital that he be inoculated with the bacilli of TB, and when they were satisfied he had cured himself, he would offer his cure to the patients free. Frederick Wood (Secretary) replied: 'The committee regret that your offer is of a nature which they are unable to accept.' Stevens had a long-running duel

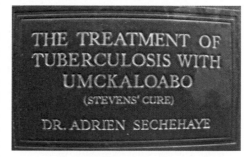

THE TREATMENT OF TUBERCULOSIS WITH UMCKALOABO
(STEVENS' CURE)

DR. ADRIEN SECHEHAYE

Figure 4 Steven's Cure 1932 (Sechehaye was a Swiss physician) (Newsom)

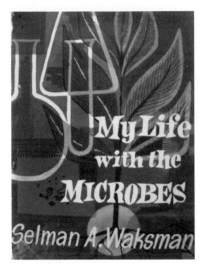

Figure 5   Waksman's autobiography (Newsom)

with the British Medical Association, starting in 1907, but the cure remained on sale until the start of the Medicines Commission. I have met one TB sufferer (proven at the Hammersmith Hospital), who took the cure as a last resort (it tasted like dog biscuits) and is now in his 90s. Umckaloabo is still on sale in Germany as a cure for respiratory tract infection, and recent work has demonstrated some anti-bacterial activity.

Things changed dramatically in 1944 with the advent of streptomycin. Selman Waksman had discovered the soil actino-mycete that produces it in 1915, but it was the approach of World War II that stimulated him to turn from soil research to antibiotic (a word he invented) research. Unlike penicillin, a chance observation, streptomycin was the result of screening perhaps 10,000 organisms.

Wakman's story is almost worth a separate article – from Russian refugee to Nobel prize-winner, but is told in his delightful book *My life with the microbes* (Waksman, 1958). He asked the US government for help with the screening programme but was told: 'We are at war, what you propose is merely of theoretical interest.'

In the end he got funds from a drug company, which when streptomycin finally appeared, graciously allowed an 'open patent' for its manufacture.

Streptomycin cured children of the dreaded TB meningitis, but had three disadvantages – resistant tubercle bacilli appeared quickly in adults (perhaps because of a larger bacterial load), it was an injection, and overdose gave toxicity.

The MRC streptomycin trial was the first properly conducted randomised drug trial ever performed (Crofton, 2006), and the MRC was heavily involved in later trials. Fortunately 'para aminosalicylic acid' was found to delay the onset of resistance, and so a streptomycin and para aminosalicylic acid (PAS) regime was introduced.

Later isoniazid was added, so that a curative mixture (provided it was given for six months or longer) became available. Even so, some patients developed resistance.

All this changed in the 1970s with the arrival of rifampicin. This replaced strep-tomycin. The new mixture was highly effective, could be taken by mouth, and was less toxic. At Papworth, one patient who had been in hospital for four years with resistant TB was suddenly cured. She was so used to 'sanatorium' life that we had to have three attempts at discharging her.

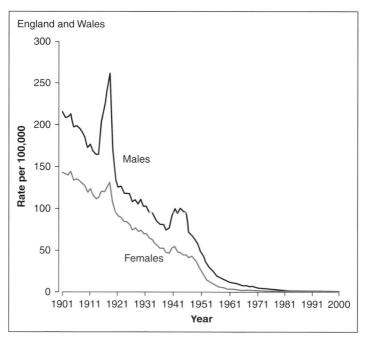

Figure 6   Government statistics on deaths from tuberculosis per 100,000 population for male and female in England and Wales (1900–2000) (PSI License C2009000939)

Finally PAS (which tasted nasty) was replaced by more powerful oral drugs, and the MRC showed that short courses (two to four months) were effective. The change from injections to tablets had one disadvantage – patient compliance. MDR and possibly XDR resistance have been encouraged by failure to take the tablets, and stimulated directly observed therapy (DOT).

Prevention

Mortality from TB in England between 1860 and 1910 fell from 3300 per million to around 1800 per million in 1900. This continued despite lack of medical intervention with two blips (especially in males) during the two world wars. Why? It reflected improved social conditions (including clean milk).

The advent of specific therapy in 1950 caused an increased decline in mortality by both treating the disease and reducing the reservoir of infection (two weeks treatment was all that was needed to render a patient non-infectious). Contact tracing with chemoprophylaxis for contacts must also have reduced the disease load.

However, the main but most controversial preventive method is BCG vaccine. Calmette and Guérin spent 13 years in the Lille Pasteur Institute (including those under German occupation in World War 1) attenuating a strain of bovine bacilli until it became 'fixed' in an avirulent state (Bacille Calmette Guérin). In 1921, after a trial in one baby (following an appeal from the family as the mother had died of TB), they began vaccinating babies in France, although no formal trial was undertaken.

Then in 1930 there was a disaster at Lubeck in Germany – 87 of 249 babies given the vaccine orally died and 80 more were ill. Investigation revealed that the vaccine had been stored in the same refrigerator as virulent tubercle bacilli.

However, the damage was done – no one trusted BCG. The final proof of its value only followed 25 years later, when an MRC trial of school children in the UK showed 85% protection after five years (Hart and Sutherland, 1977).

Even then there was controversy. In India, for example, it was less effective – perhaps because the population had already been partially immunised by other mycobacteria in their drinking water. BCG vaccination means a positive tuberculin test – so making the latter useless for contact tracing. For this reason, BCG was rarely used in the US, until the advent of MDR strains prompted its use for protecting hospital staff.

The value of the vaccine depends on the incidence of TB. My eldest son was born in Hong Kong, where one almost had to have proof of BCG vaccination before getting a birth certificate (one in seven had open TB at the time – not so now).

In the UK until recently BCG was offered to schoolchildren only after a tuberculin test. Today this is no longer felt to be cost-effective as the overall incidence of TB is so low. Nonetheless my grandson who was born in the Hammersmith Hospital in 2006 was vaccinated as he lives in an area of London where TB still occurs.

Conclusion

The history of TB suggests a success story. Certainly in the UK at present, it is so. Sadly, as we have seen, there is more to it. The advent of HIV infection with its natural immunosuppression, and the reduction in living conditions in many countries and refugee camps mean that the lessons learnt have not had their proper expression. A good summary of the current situation is given by Pratt, Grange and Williams (2005). Hopefully it is not too late to prevent the world being swamped by an epidemic of XDR.TB.

Further reading

Crofton J. (2006) The MRC randomised trial of streptomycin. *J Roy Soc Med* **99**: 531–4.
Hart PD. Sutherland I. (1977) BCG and the vole bacillus vaccines in the prevention of tuberculosis in adolescence and early adult life. Final report. *Brit Med J* **2**: 293–5.

Koch R. (1886) *The etiology of tuberculosis*: In: *Microparasites and disease.* The Sydenham Society: London: 65–200.

Lawn SD. Wilkinson R. (2006) Extensively drug resistant tuberculosis. *Brit Med J* **333**: 559–60.

Morbidity and Mortality Weekly Report. (2006) Emergence of *Mycobacterium tuberculosis* with extensive resistance to second-line drugs worldwide 2000–2004. *Morbidity and Mortality Weekly Report* **55**: 301–5.

National Collaborating Centre for Chronic Conditions. (2006) *Tuberculosis.* Royal College of Physicians: London.

Newsom SWB. (2002) Stevens cure: a secret remedy. *J Roy Soc Med* **95**: 463–7.

Pratt RJ. Grange JM. Williams VG. (2005) *Tuberculosis.* London; Hodden Arnold.

Waksman S. (1958) *My life with the microbes.* The Scientific Book Club: London.

Chapter 22

MRSA and its predecessor part 1: discovery and definition

Introduction

Fortunately for me, I retired about six months before EMRSA 14 struck in our area. However, I have had a lengthy experience of staphylococci, starting with a series of boils at the age of 15 (when penicillin was not widely used), and perhaps reaching a peak with the 'nursery outbreak' in 1959. This involved 36 babies with spots, 16 mothers with breast abscesses, and two baby deaths from pneumonia. Nonetheless staphylococci are paradoxical organisms – most of the time they are widespread and harmless. Figure 1 shows the result of a trainee nurse putting one of her hairs and prints of three fingers on a blood agar plate during a teaching session. For much of my working life nosocomial infections with gram-negative bacteria were far more important. We knew the habits of staphylococci, and anyway had coxacillin to deal with any problems.

To recap previous articles – bacteriology proper started in the 1860s with Pasteur's observations on wine, and later Lister's 'antiseptic surgery'. However,

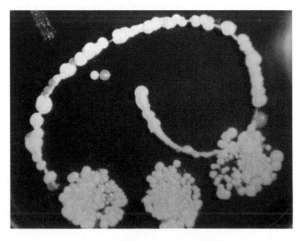

Figure 1   Growth from fingerprints and hair (Newsom)

until the development of microscopy and staining (Gram invented his stain in 1884) – no one really knew what species of bacteria were involved. As far as Lister was concerned it was the concept of germs that he attacked – and with great success. Some of the bacteria that had been seen in wound exudates as globes were called 'micrococci'. Billroth, a surgeon in Vienna described chains of cocci, and called them 'streptococci' using the Greek word for a chain.

Robert Koch did the first proper study of wound infections while he was still a GP in rural Germany. He did not have access to human material so he studied mice, which were plentiful in his barn. He transferred diseased tissue from one mouse to the next, and studied the bacteria involved. This was the first use of a microscope equipped with a condenser and an oil immersion lens, together with aniline dyes. He drew what he saw, but was unable to make further progress (he did not develop the ability to culture bacteria on solid media until 1881). In 1878 he wrote up his results in a small book, which so stimulated Lister that he had it translated by one of his assistants (Koch, 1880).

Ogston's Coccus

Alexander Ogston (1844–1929) (see Figure 2) was the first to study wound infections in humans, and it is to him we owe the name 'staphylococcus'. He had an elective in Prague, Vienna and Berlin as a medical student, and so spoke German perfectly. and had German-speaking contacts. You may have already seen his picture, as the tall surgeon with the moustache in the 'Listerian' operation in Aberdeen (see Figure 3). Ogston was a larger-than-life figure, with many facets to his life. He was a true Scot, enjoying both a house in Aberdeen and a country estate. He raised eight children, travelled a lot, and had a great interest in military medicine – so much so that he worked as a surgeon in Belgrade during the First World War in his 70s.

However, it is as an assistant surgeon in Aberdeen that he appears on the scene. Like Lister, he was devastated at the 'hospitalism' that attended surgical operations, and when he heard of the success of 'antiseptic surgery' he decided to visit Lister. The latter

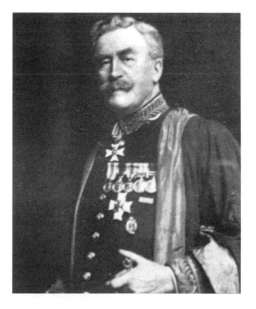

Figure 2   Sir Alexander Ogston (Wellcome Images)

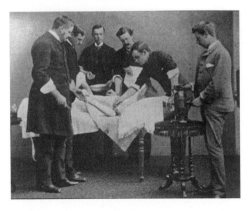

Figure 3　A 'Listerian' operation in Aberdeen (Department Surgery, Aberdeen University)

had just (1869) become a professor in Edinburgh. He writes of this in his memoirs (Ogston, 1943): I called on Lister unknown and unannounced, and was received with all the sweetness and gracious courtesy that was part of his nature.' He then went to Glasgow and saw a knee joint that had been operated on and was perfectly healed. On return to Aberdeen, he set up 'antiseptic surgery', and tore down the notice' Prepare to meet thy God' that had been over the door. Antiseptic surgery went very well in Aberdeen – the students wrote:

'The spray, the spray, the antiseptic spray,
A.O. would shower it morning, night and day.
For every sort of scratch
Where others would attach
A sticking-plaster patch
He gave the spray.'

Like all other operating surgeons Ogston asked himself: 'What is the cause of this acute suppuration occurring after wounds and operations?'. Unlike Lister, whom he found vague on this topic, he felt it must be a specific germ. One day he attended a young man called James Davidson, who had an extensive 'phlegmon' of the leg. He took some pus home and looked at it under his student microscope: 'My delight may be conceived when I saw beautiful tangles, tufts, and chains of round organisms, which stood out clear among the pus cells, all stained with the aniline violet stain I had used.' He purchased a better microscope, got a laboratory built in the garden, obtained a 'vivisection' license, and asked all his colleagues to send him pus samples.

After experimenting with culturing the pus in such surgically available liquids as urine, hydrocoele fluid, ascetic fluid or the contents of ovarian cysts in attempts to grow pure cultures, he settled on using new-laid eggs incubated at 37°C. He transferred the colonies of bacteria so obtained to another egg, until he got a single type of organism. This was then inoculated into guinea pigs or white mice. He soon found he had two types of pathogenic 'micrococci' to deal with. 'One in the form of chains or necklaces to which the name of 'streptococcus' had already been given ('I do not know by whom', he wrote), and the other growing in masses or clusters to which I gave the name 'staphylococcus'. He had asked the professor of Greek for a name, and the latter came up with staphylo – meaning a bunch of grapes. He found staphylococci in 70 'acute abscesses', and only the 14 'cold abscesses' (probably tuberculosis) he studied did not produce them.

As usual: 'The final step of convincing the medical profession of the validity of my discovery proved a rather thorny one.' The Aberdeen doctors received his ideas with incredulity. The British Medical Association (BMA) said: 'Can anything good come from Aberdeen?' Lister was encouraging, but his assistant (despite Koch's book) was very sceptical. So Ogston took the unusual step of presenting his work to an appreciative audience – namely a meeting of German surgeons in Berlin in 1880, and publishing it in Langenbeck's *Archiv fur Klinische Chirugie* under the title

'Ueber Abscesse'. The *British Medical Journal* refused to publish his later papers on the subject, so they appeared in 1882 in the *Journal of Anatomy and Physiology*. Ogston's drawings (see Figure 4) showed clearly the difference between staphylococci and streptococci and put them firmly on the map.

Ogston also realised that there might be avirulent staphylococci on the skin, and speculated on whether bacterial growth in the tissues was the source of generalised disturbances, perhaps due to ptomaines (toxins). The organisms that exist on the sur-

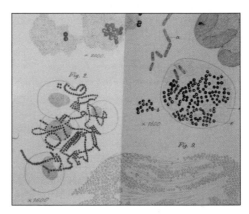

Figure 4   Ogston's drawing of streptococci and staphylococci (from Arch. Klin. Surg. 1880; 21: 588–600)

face of the skin, are they innocent or noxious?', he asked. He also connected the appearance of yellow pus, noted to be associated with severe infections, with the growth of staphylococci saying. 'In several instances, it was the deepest orange yellow.'

However, life moves on. In 1882 he was appointed Regius Professor of Surgery in Aberdeen. He wrote: 'The limited time and opportunities I possessed in the midst of a big surgical practice proved insuperable impediments, and I had to leave others… to the pursuit of further enquiries.'

Sadly Ogston had broken a rule of naming bacteria, which he certainly was unaware of – not surprisingly since it was only made in 1958 – namely that 'the name of a genus is not valid if it is not accompanied by a description of the genus or a reference to a previously published description'. Nonetheless a centenary celebration of the discovery of 'Ogston's Coccus' was held in Aberdeen in 1981 (Macdonald and Smith, 1981).

Enter Rosenbach. He was the professor extraordinary and assistant surgeon at Goettingen. Although Rosenbach worked in 1884, only a few years later, he knew of Ogston's work and that of Koch, but had the great advantage of being able to grow his bacteria on a 'peptonised meat jelly' containing agar and so see the colonies produced. From 30 'unopened abscesses', he grew five types of bacteria – far the commonest were the staphylococci ('I will here adopt the name proposed by Ogston'. he wrote (Rosenbach, 1886)). He noted two types of colony – differentiated by colour, and so called them *Staphylococcus pyogenes aureus*, and *Staphylococcus pyogenes albus*. A third colour – lemon was added later as *Staphylococcus pyogenes citreus*. It is interesting to see that the original *Staphylococcus albus* strains came from pus, and Rosenbach proved their pathogenicity in animals. Later, it was realised that most of the skin commensal bacteria were *Staphylococcus albus*, and for a while this name was used to denote harmless staphylococci. It was very inaccurate as we shall see. Rosenbach also gets the credit for the name *Streptococcus pyogenes*, because it was one of his five types.

As a footnote to all this activity one last name – Friedlander. He was the Berlin pathologist who studied pneumonia, and first isolated a gram-negative germ for which he gets no credit – we now call it Klebsiella after Dr Klebs. Friedlander it was, who employed Dr Gram to stain lungs of patients dead of pneumonia, and together they saw and described the pneumococcus. There still remained a morass of other spherical gram-positive organisms. which continued to be called 'micrococci'. Indeed it was only in the 1920s that the name 'staphylococcus' was generally used.

Diffusible products of staphylococci

For the next 50 years or so, the problems were to decide which types of staphylococci actually caused disease, and to see what the mechanisms were. Early researchers must have been heartened by the progress made with diphtheria. By 1888 the bacteria had been shown to produce a filterable toxin, and by 1895 treatment of this previously fatal disease was available in the shape of an antitoxin (an antibody made in the horse). Immunisation also was begun, by giving injections of a toxin-antitoxin mixture, which by the 1920s had been replaced by the 'toxoid' made by treating toxin with formalin to make it harmless, but still capable of stimulating an immune response. What could be done for staphylococcal infections?

Although Rosenbach had shown that 'white' staphylococci could be involved in serious infection, later workers found them mostly on skin, and indeed the name *Staphylococcus albus* was replaced by *Staphylococcus epidermidis*. Infections were usually caused by the 'golden' colonies, which became known as

Staphylococcus aureus. Much work was done to try and persuade the bacteria to produce coloured colonies, by adding chemicals to the media, or by growing at unusual temperatures. None of this worked. There was a better test around all the time – in 1903 '*Staph pyogenes*' (gold or white) was found to clot goose plasma. However, the 'coagulase test' was not really put to use for another 30 years. Then the names changed again and we had 'coagulase-positive' and 'coagulase-negative' staphylococci. Professor Elek at St George's Hospital (of whom we shall hear again) studied the relationship of coagulase and colour as seen in Figure 5, and wrote the definitive summary of *Staphylococcus pyogenes* (Elek, 1959). Nowadays, the coagulase-negative staphylococci are coming out of a 'Pandora's Box' – at the last count there were at least 30 different types (including *Staphylococcus epidermidis*). They are mainly associated with device-related infections, but that is another story.

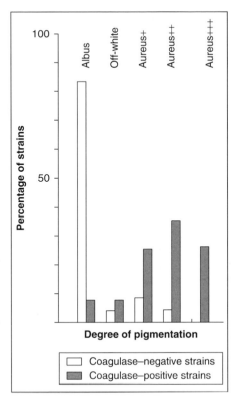

Figure 5   Correlation of coagulase production and colony colour (from Elek and Levy 1950, Br. J. Exp. Path, 31: 363)

Boils and abscesses are usually localised, so it is no surprise that pyogenic staphylococci were able to produce coagulase. They were also found to attack white blood cells – by means of a 'leucocidin'. thus encouraging pus formation. Three types of diffusible blood-destroying enzymes – the haemolysins – were found. The chief one was associated with an ability to kill rabbits, and to cause skin lesions, and was called a toxin or just staphylococcal toxin. Treating the toxin with formalin produced a staphylococcus toxoid. In the days before antibiotics, the only treatment for recurrent boils was either a vaccine of killed staphylococci, or injections of toxoid. In 1935 the standard book on vaccines said: 'Staphylococcus toxoid has been used in man to treat boils, carbuncles and other staphylococcal lesions with considerable success. The treatment is still experimental…' . I did not receive toxoid when I was 15, but later when I was a microbiology trainee in London, I used it to make a vaccine for my professor (before the Medicines Commission!).

Another toxin discovered early on was enterotoxin. The first recorded incidence of staphylococcal food poisoning involved a family eating meat from a sick cow – all but a child who had none fell ill soon afterwards, and staphylococci were grown from the partially-cooked meat – in 1894. Enterotoxin causes sickness within a few hours. Fortunately what comes quickly goes quickly too, and sufferers should be better within 48 hours.

Addendum

Recent interest has been shown in another toxin – the Panton-Valentine leucocidin. Panton and Valentine working in London demonstrated a toxin that only acted on human (as opposed to other species) white blood cells. Their results were reported in the *Lancet* in 1932, but only recently has there been enough interest in PVL producing *Staph aureus* strains (PVL-SA) to warrant the HPA document: Guidance on the diagnosis and management of PVL-associated *Staphylococcus aureus* (PVL-SA) infections in England (2008) (I should know about this as I edited it!!!). An associated problem also to appear is the Community-acquired MRSA – but fortunately for me this is a current rather than historic event.

Conclusion

This article has considered the definition of *Staphylococcus aureus,* and some of its chief properties. In Part 2 another Scottish doctor called Alexander will appear, and clinical manifestations, antibiotics and epidemiology will be discussed.

Further reading

Elek SD. (1959) *Staphylococcus pyogenes and its relation to disease.* Livingstone: Edinburgh and London.

Koch R. (1880) *Investigations Into the etiology of traumatic infective diseases.* Watson Cheyne W. (Transl.) New Sydenham Society: London.

Macdonald A. Smith C. (Eds.). (1981) *The Staphylococci: proceedings of the Alexander Ogston Centennial Conference.* Aberdeen University Press: Aberdeen.

Newsom SWB. (2008) Ogston's Coccus. *Journal of Hospital Infection*; 70: 369–72

Ogston WH. (1943) *Alexander Ogston KCVO.* Aberdeen University Press: Aberdeen.

Rosenbach FJ. (1886) Suppuration and septic diseases. In: Watson Cheyne W. (Ed.). *Recent essays on bacteria in relation to disease.* New Sydenham Society: London.

Chapter 23

MRSA and its predecessor part 2: infections, outbreaks, and the advent of penicillin

---

Introduction

Staphylococci is such a big topic – historically, as well as today (Duckworth, 2003) – that I have split it into three parts.

In the previous chapter we learnt how Alexander Ogston defined staphylococci and set the scene by noting that some strains were not pathogenic, and asking what toxins (he called them 'ptomaines') were involved. Rosenbach got credit for the name and described both golden (aureus) and white (albus) colonies, although both types had been isolated from clinical lesions. Later, the disease-producers were all shown to clot plasma, and hence were called: 'coagulase-positive'. As we now use terms such as MRSA and methicillin-sensitive *Staphylococcus aureus* (MSSA) for the methicillin-resistant, and methicillin susceptible strains of *Staphylococcus aureus* – I will call all the coagulase-positive, potentially pathogenic strains by this name.

Clinical picture

Staphylococcal coagulase can be thought of as forming a clot around the bacteria, thus localising their effect and protecting them as they grow, while leucocidin could explain pus formation. Hence, localised skin lesions are the commonest staphylococcal infections – boils, abscesses, carbuncles, styes, and whitlows – all on the skin. My recurrent boils came when I was 'run down' – a rapidly-growing adolescent who had just finished 'O' levels. Several diseases predispose to staphylococcal infection. Diabetes is the main one (finding a growth of *Staphylococcus aureus* in urine is often a marker for diabetes), but influenza may be followed by staphylococcal pneumonia – a worry with the swine flu pandemic, and cystic fibrosis predisposes to infection in the bronchi. Injecting drug addicts are susceptible to deep seated infections, especially endocarditis affecting the right side of the heart.

Staphylococcal septicaemia is quite common. An up-to-date study from Jerusalem showed that *Staphylococcus aureus* was found in 1,240 out of 173,571 (0.71%) blood cultures, second only to *E. coli*. Once in the body staphylococci can cause deep-seated abscesses – especially in the kidney, and sometimes in muscle, together with septic arthritis and osteomyelitis. The biggest killer, however, is endocarditis.

Staphylococcal toxaemia is quite rare – apart from enterotoxin (see Chapter 22) – the other main toxic diseases include the 'toxic shock' syndrome, and the 'scalded skin' syndrome. One last illness, rarely seen today but a warning of things to come, was the enterocolitis that followed treatment with broad-spectrum antibiotics in the 1950s. This was long before *Clostridium difficile* colitis, but treatment was the same – oral vancomycin. It was thought to be due to staphylococci, and indeed a simple diagnosis could be made by looking with the unaided eye at a gram-stained film of faeces: it was blue and contained sheets of staphylococci. Vancomycin certainly worked, but later workers think that this was really a *Clostridium difficile* problem all the time.

Three illustrative cases

Three patients with endocarditis demonstrate the problems of staphylococcal infections.

Case 1

The first case was of a 12-year-old boy, known to have a heart murmur, who came

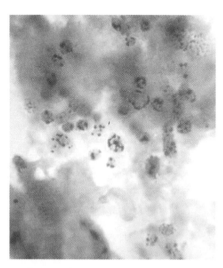

home from school feeling 'flu-ish'. During the week that followed he developed headache, fever, and a sore knee, and saw three separate general practitioners. The first two said: 'Flu', and prescribed aspirin. The third sent him into hospital with a diagnosis of 'viral infection'. Next day, the blood cultures grew a heavy growth of *Staphylococcus aureus*, which was also present in his urine, and staphylococci could actually be seen in a normal blood film. When I went to the ward with the results I found the cardiac team already there. He had endocarditis, and by the end of the week (only two weeks after first feeling ill) his aortic valve was completely destroyed and he required an emergency valve replacement (Figure 1 shows a Gram-stained

Figure 1   Gram's stain of impression from a heart valve showing staphylococcal endocarditis (Newsom)

film of a smear from his valve). It was successful despite his renal failure. Sadly, the damage to his heart was too great and he died some months later. The most likely source of his infection was the staphylococci in his nose. He had had a nose bleed two days before he fell ill.

Case 2

Next, is the case of a middle-aged general practitioner with psoriasis. He had a stressful life, and occasionally took it out on his skin. He was admitted to Papworth with staphylococcal endocarditis, and after antibiotic treatment had a valve replacement. Some years later the stress reoccurred and he had a second bout of endocarditis – this time on the prosthetic valve, caused by the identical strain of *staphylococcus* (it was erythromycin-resistant). The valve was replaced, but three years later the same problem recurred, although this time antibiotics alone were successful. I wanted to give him a bedside box of flucloxacillin to take whenever he felt stressed, but the consensus was that he should take it regularly for life – and indeed this prevented any further infections.

Case 3

The last example arrived for a heart transplant from a hospital where an MRSA epidemic was under way (it was not around in Papworth at the time). We were told that this patient had not been in touch with any MRSA patients, and had proved negative on screening. Nonetheless, within four days of the operation his screening cultures grew MRSA. His post-operative progress was uneventful, apart from the problems of isolation. However, two years later he returned with cardiac complications. Once again he came from the previous hospital – with a clean bill of health as regards MRSA. Once again we grew the same strain of MRSA; however, this time it came from a blood culture, and his infection proved fatal.

The first case demonstrates how a local lesion (nosebleed) can let in the germs. Progression of the illness, which often resembles 'flu' in its early stages, can be frighteningly quick, in this case his heart and kidneys had been involved before he entered hospital. The second patient shows how seemingly benignly diseased skin can harbour large numbers of staphylococci, which despite all our efforts with Hibiscrub baths and local treatment can persist for years. The last patient occurred in the mupirocin era, and twice was said to be free from MRSA after standard screening, but clearly was not. He also showed that MRSA was not, as some thought at the time, less pathogenic than MSSA, and can be extremely difficult to eradicate, and to be sure of eradication.

Antibiotics 1

Sulphonamides were the first successful antimicrobial agents to be used (in the 1930s – I know because M&B 693 cured my brucellosis). However, they had little effect on staphylococci in the human, as they were neutralised by pus. Enter the second Alexander, Alexander Fleming (Figure 2), Scottish but working in

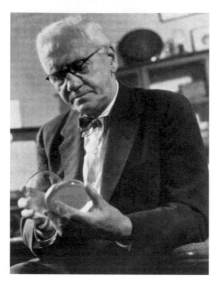

Figure 2　Sir Alexander Fleming (Wellcome Images)

London, where his chance finding of a culture plate contaminated with *Penicillium notatum* in 1928 initiated the 'antibiotic era'. He wrote: 'Such contamination is usually regarded as a reflection on the technique of the bacteriologist'. 'This plate had to be opened for examination under a microscope, and then left for further observation. The mould developed into a large colony. This in itself did not call for comment, but what was surprising was that the staphylococcal colonies in the neighbourhood of the mould that had been well developed were observed now to be showing signs of dissolution' (Fleming, 1946). Thus the start of penicillin, which did indeed prove most effective for treating staphylococcal infection – particularly in wounded soldiers.

Penicillin works by stopping bacteria building new cell wall components, which they need to coat and protect growing bacteria. There are two perfectly normal ways bacteria (staphylococci included) can avoid a subsequent death from exposure to penicillin. The first is by not growing. When say 1000 bacteria are exposed to a killing dose of penicillin – most die quickly, but some cells live for another two and a half days; they 'persist', presumably because they are not growing. The second way is illustrated

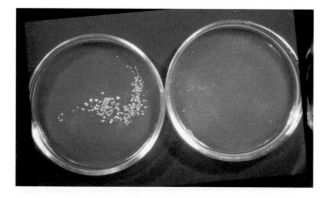

Figure 3　Cultures of pus from a woman receiving flucloxacillin. The left hand plate has had sugar added to the growth medium, so damaged bacteria are still able to grow. (Newsom)

in Figure 3, which shows two plates which had been filled with the nutrient agar, each inoculated with a drop of pus from a patient whose empyema was not responding to cloxacillin. The only difference was that the left-hand plate contained extra sugar. This provided a stable environment for bacteria whose cell walls were deficient, but as you can see were still alive. Most times this 'persistence' does not matter, as the normal body defences can cope.

Fleming had noted that not all bacteria were susceptible to penicillin. Gram-negative bacilli such as *E. coli* were resistant, and by 1945 workers in Oxford had shown that these produced an enzyme, which they called 'penicillinase'. Some staphylococci also produced penicillinase. There was a race between the penicillin trying to kill the bacteria, and the bacterial enzymes destroying the penicillin. This is illustrated in Figure 4, which shows a plate containing blood agar. Two sides have been cut away and replaced with penicillin containing agar. Bacteria have been streaked across the plate, a fully penicillin-susceptible staphylococcus in the centre, and a penicillin-resistant strain on the outer sides. The intermediate streaks were from a dilution of the resistant strain. The resistant strain grows very well, even on top of the penicillin agar. When diluted the strain has been set back a bit, while the susceptible strain has almost been wiped out.

Epidemiology

In the 1950s came a gradual rise of the penicillin-resistant 'hospital staphylococcus'. The strains gradually developed resistance to other antibiotics, notably erythromycin and tetracycline, and became the commonest staphylococci in

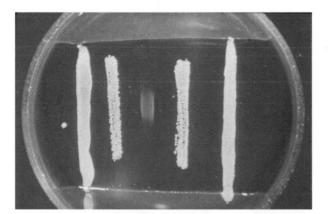

Figure 4   A culture plate filled with blood agar, the top and bottom of which has been replaced by clear agar containing penicillin. The central streak is a penicillin-susceptible staphylococcus. The other streaks are of the same penicillin-resistant strain. The inner streaks are from a 1/1000 dilution of the original culture – so did not make enough penicillinase in time, and were more susceptible to the penicillin (Newsom)

hospitals. My successor as house physician nearly died from staphylococcal pneumonia after performing mouth-to-mouth resuscitation on a dying patient. The last available antibiotic worked, but it was touch and go, since at least three others failed.

Where had they come from? Some penicillin resistant staphylococci were later found in nose swabs from aborigines in New Guinea who had never been exposed to other tribes of humans, never mind antibiotics. There must have been some other reason for developing the ability to produce penicillinase (Rountree, 1956). By now it was possible to read the labels on strains of staphylococci by bacteriophage typing, which involves establishing a pattern of susceptibility to a standard set of bacteriophages. The strain of staphylococcus under test is dried onto an agar plate, which is then overlaid with a set of drops containing the different phages, some of which may destroy the bacteria, so generating a pattern or bacteriophage type (see Figure 5). Penicillin-resistant strains were of different phage types to the susceptible strains, which remained commonest in the community. The resistant strains occurred in staff who had never received penicillin therapy; as early as 1947, 37% of strains isolated at St Thomas' Hospital were penicillin-resistant. In those days penicillin was given by injection. People would expel air from a loaded syringe before giving an injection, and penicillin was found in ward air by Dr Gould in Edinburgh. It is not surprising that staff inhaled enough to kill their original penicillin-susceptible staphylococci and allow the 'hospital' germs to replace them. Healthy workers in penicillin manufacturing plants also carried resistant strains. Nurse's uniforms at St Bartholomew's Hospital were found to be contaminated with staphylococci, so providing another route of spread.

The 'nursery' outbreak I described in Chapter 22 occurred in our London Hospital in 1958; other smaller outbreaks had occurred on the surgical wards, but the nursery provided the largest problem. I still have my notebook containing the results of my investigations (no ICNs then), and the paper I wrote (in the *Medical School Clinical Supplement*) described our findings. Nearly all the clinical lesions (breast abscesses, spotty babies) were caused by the phage Type 80 staphylococcus, which I also found on blankets, nappy trolleys and scales in the nursery; but of course the real (but unwitting) culprit was the midwife who had a boil on her finger.

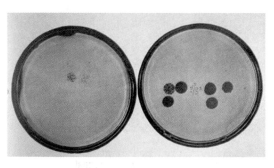

Figure 5   Bacteriophage typing of staphylococci (Newsom)

Type 80 (later type 80/81) had an interesting history – it was first described in Sydney, Australia in 1953 (Rountree, 1960) – see Figure 6. This was long before the days of mass jet travel, and Australia was a far away place. Type 80 arrived in Southampton in 1957, and within the year had caused 30% of all outbreaks in England; with a particular predilection for nurseries (in those days babies routinely stayed in a nursery for ten days or so). If a patient turned up in casualty with a serious staphylococcal infection – the question to ask was – Have you a new baby in the house? Surprisingly, often the answer was: 'Yes'.

So at the end of the 1950s staphylococcal infection could be very worrying. Even in 1966 the standard text *Hospital infection* by Williams, Blowers, Garrod and Shooter (1966), concentrated much more on staphylococcal problems than it did on the gram-negative bacteria. Post-operative surgical sepsis led to concentration on operating theatres. The ventilation of St Bartholomew's, for

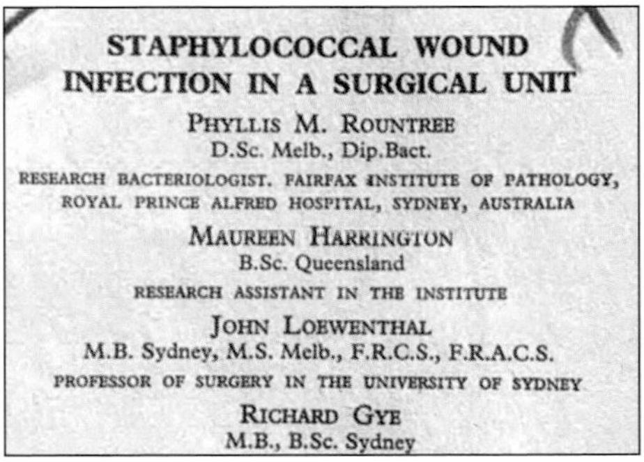

STAPHYLOCOCCAL WOUND INFECTION IN A SURGICAL UNIT

PHYLLIS M. ROUNTREE
D.Sc. Melb., Dip.Bact.
RESEARCH BACTERIOLOGIST, FAIRFAX INSTITUTE OF PATHOLOGY,
ROYAL PRINCE ALFRED HOSPITAL, SYDNEY, AUSTRALIA

MAUREEN HARRINGTON
B.Sc. Queensland
RESEARCH ASSISTANT IN THE INSTITUTE

JOHN LOEWENTHAL
M.B. Sydney, M.S. Melb., F.R.C.S., F.R.A.C.S.
PROFESSOR OF SURGERY IN THE UNIVERSITY OF SYDNEY

RICHARD GYE
M.B., B.Sc. Sydney

Figure 6   News from Australia – 1960

example, was shown to carry staphylococci from the wards into the theatre – a good stimulus for closing the windows and having positive pressure ventilation in theatres. Blowers studied the paradox of the healthy staphylococcal carrier, showing that carriage was probably not as important as the ability of a few people to 'disperse' large numbers of bacteria into the air. Skin lesions, even those not obviously infected, can, however, become heavily colonised with staphylococci, and if on the hands can be especially dangerous.

Antibiotics 2

The last-ditch antibiotic of the time was 'Vancomycin' (I vanquish). This had only been discovered in 1956, but so desperate was the need for therapy for staphylococcal infections that the US Food and Drugs Administration granted a licence in 1958 – is this a record? The original datasheet (Figure 7 shows the cover) was typewritten and refers to a product with 82% purity. What was the other 18%? Well the brown colour prompted the name of 'Mississippi mud'. The molecular structure and mode of action were unknown, and the molecular weight was stated as twice what it actually turned out to be. The product was (not unexpectedly) fairly toxic – infusions often caused phlebitis and both renal- and ototoxicity were common – but it worked. It was a life-saver. Today, despite its

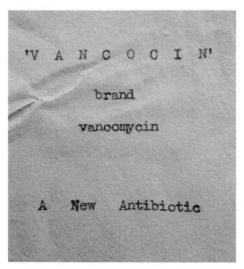

'V A N C O C I N'

brand

vancomycin

A New Antibiotic

Figure 7   Vancomycin – the original datasheet
(Newsom)

age, Vancomycin has had a renaissance – more on this in the next chapter. Suffice to say that it is now purer/less toxic, and its mode of action is fully understood. It is more rapidly bactericidal than a B-lactam drug, and as a child of the 1950s I always remembered to use it as my last-ditch for overwhelming infection – for example, in the 12-year-old boy (page 188) after previous therapy had failed.

I hope I have painted a fairly desperate picture – perhaps even worse than the current rampaging of the MRSA. Even in 1955 *The Lancet* printed an editorial on: The unconquered staphylococcus (Anon, 1955).

Further reading

Anon. (1955) The unconquered staphylococcus. *Lancet* **ii**: 755–6.

Duckworth G. (2003) Controlling methicillin-resistant *Staphylococcus aureus*. *BMJ* **327**: 1177–8.

Fleming A. (Ed.). (1946) *Penicillin – its practical application*. Butterworth: London. (The history of penicillin is presented here).

Rountree PM. (1956) Staphylococci harboured by people in Western Highlands of New Guinea. *Lancet* **i**: 719–20.

Rountree PM. Harrington M. Loewenthal J. Gye R. (1960) Staphylococcal infection in a surgical unit. *Lancet* **ii**: 1–6.

Williams REO. Blowers R. Garrod LP. Shooter RA. (1966) *Hospital infection, causes and prevention*. Lloyd-Luke: London.

Chapter 24
MRSA and its predecessor part 3: the rise of MRSA and EMRSA

Introduction

My last article ended in 1960 with a fairly desperate picture – perhaps even worse than the current rampaging of MRSA, but from 1960 to 1990 my reaction to therapy of staphylococcal infection was smug – I knew all about it, and gram-negative bacteria were a greater problem.

Antibiotics 3

The reason for regarding the problem as solved was the introduction of methicillin, followed shortly by cloxacillin and then flucloxacillin. How did this arise? When the NHS was being planned in the 1940s, Beechams (now part of Glaxo-SmithKlineBeechams) decided to move from manufacturing patent medicines (for example, Beechams' Pills, Veno's Cough Cure) to prescription medicines. A new research laboratory was opened at Brockham Park by Sir Alexander Fleming, whose shadow certainly hovered over it. In May 1957 the Beechams research team isolated the penicillin nucleus 6-aminopenicillanic acid (6-APA). This had very little antibacterial activity, but was readily modifiable by adding chemicals, thus forming the basis for 'semi-synthetic' penicillins. The team did not realise the full value of their discovery, and once again the *British Medical Journal* got it wrong: 'this was of uncertain value' they wrote. Nowadays, 11,000 tonnes of 6-APA are made each year.

Things moved very quickly, staphylococci were resistant to penicillin because they produced an enzyme that destroyed it. Penicillin has the molecular structure shown in Figure 1a. The 'penicillinase' enzyme was shown to act on the central square – which is a ß-lactam ring – so the enzyme became known as a ß-lactamase. Methicillin, which was the second semi-synthetic penicillin was made from 6-APA (Figure 1b) by modification of the left hand 'benzyl' ring by addition of two methoxy arms (OCH_3). These physically enfolded the ß–lactam ring and protected it from the ß-lactamase. Methicillin was marketed with great enthusiasm in

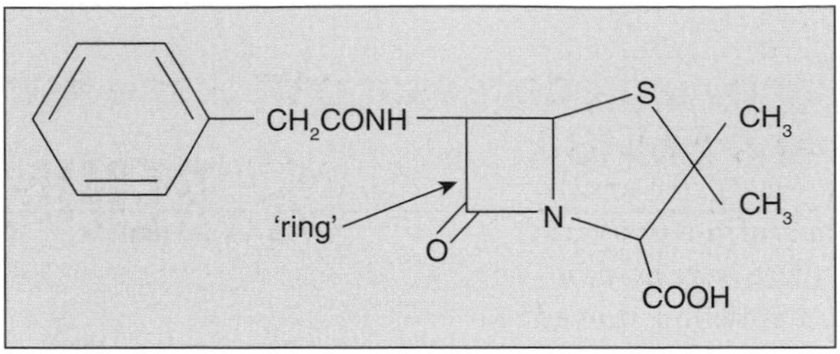

Figure 1a   Benzylpenicillin molecule (the ring is a ß–lactam ring)

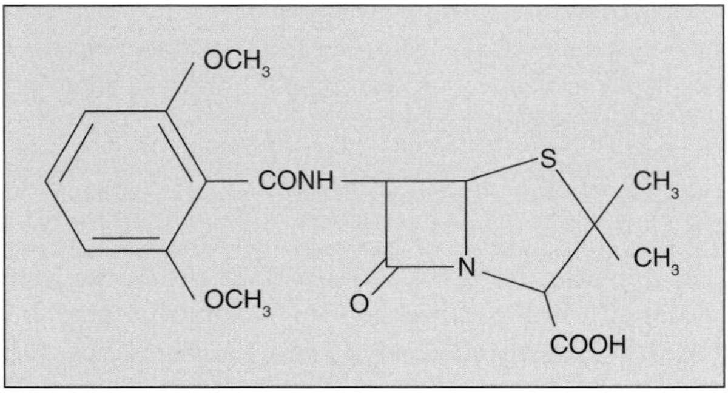

Figure 1b   Dimethoxybenzylpenicilllin (methicillin)

September 1960, see Figure 2 – the name Celbenin came from the initials of CEL Bencard, one of Beechams' executives. Like cloxacillin, its successor, it had a narrow spectrum of activity – really just the penicillin-resistant staphylococci (despite the advertisement's claim of 'active against the usual penicillin-sensitive microorganisms'). Its big disadvantage was its need for intramuscular or intravenous injections. Nonetheless, the arrival of a non-toxic and efficient cure for staphylococcal infection was a major event in chemotherapy. *The Lancet* (Rolinson, 1960; Anon, 1960) carried three papers and an editorial to introduce methicillin on 10 September 1960.

In January 1961 two papers were published describing methicillin-resistance. The first involved laboratory artefacts – cultures trained on gradually increasing concentrations of drug in the Hammersmith Hospital. Perhaps more relevant were the three strains sent from an anonymous hospital to Colindale for bacteriophage typing, and documented by Dr Patricia Jevons (Jevons, 1961), who thereby earned her place as a 'pioneer'. At the time,

methicillin had only been prescribed once in the hospital –
for a diabetic with boils, who
was unrelated to the patients
who grew the three strains.
However, apart from this early
warning – there were no problems, and methicillin proved
an excellent drug. Vancomycin
usage plummeted. In 1962
Beechams introduced a variant
of methicillin with an extra
chlorine atom – Cloxacillin –
which could be given by mouth
and was more potent and less
toxic. This was later supplemented by flucloxacillin (with
a fluorine atom in addition to
the chlorine). Flucloxacillin
was said to be better absorbed
from the gut. For a time there

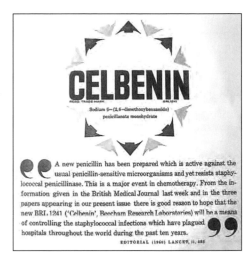

Figure 2   Advertising Methicillin in 1960 (The Chemist and Druggist)

was a price war between the two; whichever was in favour accounted for the
greatest cost in our Cambridge hospital antibiotics bill in the early 1980s.
These two new drugs meant there was no longer any need for methicillin, and
it was withdrawn from sale.

So why are MRSA so called when methicillin is not used, in fact, no longer
even made? Laboratory tests showed that special conditions were needed for
accurate laboratory tests of staphylococcal susceptibility to methicillin (and
clox/flucloxacillin). The resistance was 'heterogenous' – i.e. affected only a few
of the bacteria in a culture – so might be missed on normal susceptibility tests.
By the 1970s a reliable test was introduced – using a methicillin disc. Not long
after the test was instituted in our Papworth laboratory we had a mini-outbreak
involving four patients in adjacent beds. It was safely contained, but where had
it come from? When I telephoned the referring hospital of the index patient, the
pathologist (no microbiologists or infection control nurses there then) said:
'I think we are doing the new tests, I'll go and look'. When he investigated – he
found an (unknown to him) outbreak on the orthopaedic ward, which had been
there for some time.

Long after it had been withdrawn from sale for patients, methicillin remained
in use for the laboratory tests, and the germs continued being called MRSA, but
today, as methicillin is no longer available, oxacillin discs are used instead. For

some unaccountable reason the name methicillin (which related to those OCH_3-methoxy groups) is now changed to meticillin. Fortunately MRSA remains MRSA.

Epidemiology – 2

One of the papers in the 1960 *Lancet* came from St George's Hospital (Figure 3), where nursery infections had been a problem. The authors had obtained trial supplies of methicillin even before it went on sale, and following the work of Gould (Chapter 23), they sprayed methicillin into the nursery air. Four grams of drug per day diluted in 20ml of water were sprayed with a small hand spray gun. The newborn babies were indeed protected from 'hospital staphylococci'. The authors tried to develop methicillin-resistant strains in the laboratory, but were unable to do so. They concluded that this was a simple way to prevent spread of the 'hospital' staphylococcus and recommended it as a basis for further research.

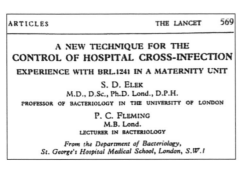

ARTICLES   THE LANCET   569

A NEW TECHNIQUE FOR THE
CONTROL OF HOSPITAL CROSS-INFECTION
EXPERIENCE WITH BRL.1241 IN A MATERNITY UNIT

S. D. ELEK
M.D., D.Sc., Ph.D. Lond., D.P.H.
PROFESSOR OF BACTERIOLOGY IN THE UNIVERSITY OF LONDON

P. C. FLEMING
M.B. Lond.
LECTURER IN BACTERIOLOGY

*From the Department of Bacteriology,
St. George's Hospital Medical School, London, S.W.1*

Figure 3   St George's *Lancet* paper

The St George's paper created considerable interest at a time when 'fogging' of rooms with disinfectants was already practised – perhaps a continuation of the 'fumigation' of my youth. For a while, I used a phenolic disinfectant spray for terminal disinfection of rooms used for barrier nursing. In the same year an infection control team in Melbourne reported on: 'spraying chlorhexidine into the ward air regularly to reduce environmental contamination with staphylococci', noting that a 'thrice-daily fogging with 1/1000 hibitane caused no inconvenience to patients'. These workers clearly later took note of the St George's paper. An Australian infectious disease consultant, a medical student in Melbourne in the 1960s, remembers asking the microbiologist what was he doing with that 'funny' box on the surgical wards? 'Preventing cross-infection with my methicillin spray' came the reply.

And so in the 1960s the Type 80 had lost its sting, and we felt secure in the knowledge that we had staphylococci under control. Occasional isolates of MRSA were made – but these were usually fully susceptible to other antibiotics and not a problem. There was even doubt as to their ability to cause disease. Some strains were reported from countries such as Poland, Turkey and India, where methicillin/cloxacillin was not available. Resistance mechanisms were studied, and it was found that MRSA had an extra cell wall protein, one that was not affected by methicillin and allowed the bacteria to build cell walls normally. The original protein was PBP2 (penicillin-binding-protein2[of 3]), and the new one was called PBP2' (prime). Later, the geneticists found a gene mecA which specified the manufacture of PBP2'. Its discovery allowed an alternative method for susceptibility testing of staphylococci, i.e. testing for presence of the gene.

Most of the interest was centred in Europe. In 1967 the first case was reported in the US. This was a laboratory-acquired infection in a scientist who jabbed his finger while making a subculture of a strain sent from France. Cellulitis developed rapidly and he required vancomycin therapy. The incident was instructive because it refuted claims that MRSA was avirulent, and provided another example of the danger of sending dangerous germs around the world. Methicillin susceptibility tests were not introduced into the US for some years – so there may have been some false confidence there – (at any rate today's incidence of MRSA in the US equals that elsewhere).

The Lancet editorial (Anon, 1960) had given an early warning: 'we must repeat that no drug or combination of drugs is ever likely to make hospitals safe for patients unless it is used in a more responsible manner than has been usual since antibiotics became available. Aseptic methods will have to be better understood and faithfully practised'. Prophetic words: the scene changed in the mid-1970s. The first reports were from Victoria in Australia, where MRSA had already been found, but accounted for <2% of isolates before 1975. By 1979, however, the State Health Commission was alarmed enough to send a questionnaire to all hospitals asking about the incidence of MRSA (defined as number of new patients harbouring the germ). More than 2,500 patients in Melbourne were known to be infected or colonised, and MRSA accounted for 20–40% of all staphylococcal isolates in the six teaching hospitals. Figure 4 charts the position in one teaching hospital – showing how the presence of an isolation ward helped, but failed when the number of beds became inadequate. In May 1982 the problem had widened to the extent that the *Medical Journal of Australia* devoted a whole issue to it (*Medical Journal of Australia*, 1982). These strains were now resistant to many different antibiotics, and vancomycin came into its own again. The pathogenicity of these strains was not in doubt. In 1981 one of the Melbourne teaching hospitals reported that 50% of all staphylococcal isolates were methicillin-resistant. Out of the 545 culture–positive patients, 254 had clinically significant infections and 75 died.

During the 1980s other epidemics of nosocomial infection were reported, and Dublin appeared to have an ongoing problem. In 1986 Ayliffe et al, noted in the Introduction to the 'guidelines' (see below): 'The situation in London and other parts of south-east England is such that at least 12 major hospitals have continuing problems with MRSA'. A notable feature of the strains involved was the ease with which they spread. A new name EMRSA (for Epidemic MRSA) was coined. The

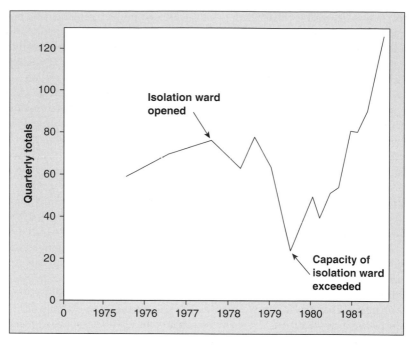

Figure 4   MRSA in a Melbourne Hospital (1982) (*Medical Journal of Australia*)

Australians got pride of place with EMRSA-1. A new molecular typing system – pulsed field gel electrophoresis – was introduced to complement bacteriophage typing for labelling the epidemic strains of MRSA. The situation required a national approach and a working party from the Hospital Infection Society and the British Society for Antimicrobial Chemotherapy was assembled to produce guidelines for control of EMRSA. These were published in the *Journal of Hospital Infection* in 1985, and a revised version was published in 1990.

The role of topical agents for decontamination of carriers was stressed in the guidelines, together with the need for hand care. Mupirocin was much used for nasal carriers. Sadly, today mupirocin-resistance is quite common, and overall success in elimination of nasal carriage may be as low as 50%. An interesting and equally effective alternative – has been reported in a paper in the *Journal of Hospital Infection* – namely tea tree oil.

The role of antiseptics in handwashing in relation to MRSA has also been queried. In 1985 I reported in an earlier version of the *Journal of Infection Control Nursing* (a supplement to the *Nursing Times*) on a simple test for persistence of antibacterial activity on surgeons' hands during an operation following scrubbing-up with 4% chlorhexidine. Gloves were worn for six hours, removed, and then a palm print was made by the surgeon onto a 10-inch square assay dish, filled with nutrient agar. The plate was then returned to the laboratory and layered with 80ml of agar containing 1ml of an 18-hour culture of *Staphylococcus epidermidis.* Figure 5 shows the outcome. I had identical results when a plate was layered with an MRSA culture.

Fortunately, Melbourne and even London was still far enough away from rural Cambridgeshire, for only occasional isolates of MRSA to be made at Papworth. However, our situation changed dramatically in 1991, when nearby Kettering was struck by a large outbreak of nosocomial infection with a new type of MRSA – EMRSA-16, which involved at least 400 patients with spread into the community. The heroic attempts to contain this were well written up by Cox and her colleagues (Cox et al, 1995a; Cox et al, 1995b) in the *Journal of Hospital Infection* in 1995. By then the wheel had turned full circle and the Cambridge antibiotics bill was headed by vancomycin (also used for *Clostridium difficile* colitis). Fortunately for me, I retired soon afterwards, and so this personal history ceases. However I was able to meet old friends and re-live our experiences at the Wellcome Witness Seminar on 'Superdrugs and Superbugs' in 2006, sometime after these articles were written. The transcript of the afternoon is now available for £6 from the Wellcome Trust at UCL (see below), and makes good reading for those into history of MRSA. The transcript Introduction was written by Professor David Greenwood, whose own delightful book on Antimicrobial Drugs is essential reading for all interested in the history of medicine, albeit rather more costly.

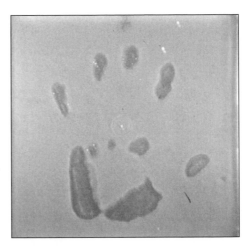

Figure 5   Palm print on staphylococcal culture plate showing persistence of antibacterial activity after washing with chlorhexidine (Newsom)

Current status

The problem persists. Figure 6 shows a comparison of the number of papers thrown up by entering MRSA into the Pubmed database. Books have been written on the topic – for example, *Methicillin-resistant Staphylococcus aureus* by Mary McCafferkey in Dublin (McCafferkey (ed), 1992). I have only given you a few key references, it is impossible to do full justice to the literature in a short history.

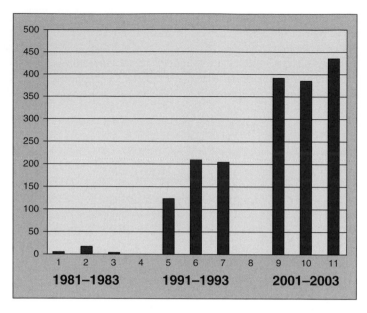

Figure 6   Comparison of numbers of papers on staphylococci printed in the 1980s/1990s/2000s (Newsom)

A revised version of the UK guidelines from a working party, strengthened by inclusion of ICNA (IPS) members, is in operation, with which you are undoubtedly familiar. Opinions vary from a 'search and destroy' approach (favoured by Cox (1995a)) to: 'efforts to control spread of EMRSA are counterproductive, and energies should be directed to outbreaks of the disease, and preventing emergence of antibiotic resistance' (Barrett, 1998) – this has produced a lively debate.

A recent (sadly not the 'last') word comes from Dr Georgia Duckworth at the Communicable Disease Surveillance Centre (CDSC), who was responsible for drafting the UK guidelines, in an editorial in the *British Medical Journal* (Duckworth, 2003). She notes that MRSA now account for 42% of all reported staphylococcal bacteraemias in the UK, the highest rate in Europe. EMRSA-1, which probably came from Australia to London in the 1980s, has now been replaced by EMRSA-15 and 16. While vancomycin remains the mainstay of treatment, some newer agents have been used, and both intermediate and full resistance to vancomycin have now been described. Although the main problems of MRSA have been in bacteraemias and wound infections, leucocidin-producing strains have been involved in serious skin infections, and in necrotising pneumonia in the community. MRSA-associated toxic shock syndrome has occurred. While most MRSA problems are hospital-based, Dr Duckworth notes several papers recording community-acquired infections, and mentions the well known problem of long-term care homes in which the elderly are at risk, and for which further guidelines have been drawn up. She concludes with a vigorous defence of 'search and destroy', which in the light of recent Government support for infection control initiatives has the chance of being better supported than before. Finally – watch out for new guidelines – the MRSA working party has been reconvened.

Further reading

Anon. (1960) Penicillinase-resistant penicillins. *Lancet* **ii**: 585–6.

Barrett SP. Mummery SV. Chattopadhyay. (1998) Trying to control MRSA causes more problems than it solves. *Journal of Hospital Infection* **39**: 85–93.

Cox RA. Conquest C. Mallaghan C. Marples RR. (1995a) A major outbreak of methicillin resistant Staphylococcus aureus caused by a new phage-type (EMRSA-16). *Journal of Hospital Infection* **29**: 87–106.

Cox RA. Mallaghan C. Conquest C. King J. (1995b) Epidemic methicillin-resistant Staphylococcus aureus: controlling the spread outside hospital. *Journal of Hospital Infection* **29**: 107–19.

Dryden M. Dailly S. Crouch M. (2004) A randomized controlled trial of Tea tree topical preparations versus a standard topical regimen for the clearance of MRSA colonization. *Journal of Hospital Infection;* **56**: 283–6.

Duckworth G. (2003) Controlling methicillin resistant Staphylococcus aureus. *British Medical Journal* **327**: 1177–8.

Greenwood D. (2008) *Antimicrobial Drugs: chronicle of a twentieth century triumph.* Oxford, Oxford University Press.

Jevons MP. (1961) 'Celbenin'-resistant staphylococci. *British Medical Journal* **i**: 124–5.

McCafferkey M. (ed) (1992) *Methicillin-resistant Staphylococcus aureus.* Marcel Decker: New York.

Medical Journal of Australia (1982) **i**: 11. Methicillin-resistant Staphylococcus aureus. (whole issue devoted to this topic).

Reynolds LA. Tansey EM. (2008) *Superbugs and superdrugs: A history of MRSA.* London: The Wellcome Trust.

Rolinson GL. Stevens S. Batchelor FR. Cameron Wood J. Chain EB. (1960) Bacteriological studies on a new penicillin – BRL 1241. *Lancet* **ii**: 564–9.

Chapter 25
Serratia marcescens: A colourful microbe

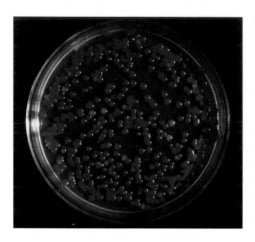

Figure 1   Culture of *Serratia marcescens*

Introduction

'Newsom', said the professor, 'I want you to test this surgeon's mask'. 'Go to the roof garden, gargle with a broth culture of *Chromobacterium prodigiosum*, put the mask on and read aloud for ten minutes holding an agar plate in front of your mouth'. I thoroughly enjoyed escaping from the laboratory to the Westminster Medical School roof garden with its view of the Houses of Parliament. Today I would think twice about swallowing that culture, as we recognise *Serratia marcescens* as an antibiotic-resistant pathogen, capable of causing nosocomial infections. However its ability to produce a red pigment (prodigiosin) makes it a good marker germ (Figure 1), and growth on starchy foods means its effects have been recognised since medieval times. Today we call it a 'coliform' and link it with klebsiellas and enterobacters. Pigment is not produced by all strains, and laboratory subcultures may lose the ability to make it, so that colonies resemble those of other coliforms. It has been isolated from water, soil, sewerage, foodstuffs and animals. There are two excellent historical reviews one from Gaughren in 1969 and the other by Yu in 1979, from which I have quoted extensively.

The bleeding bread

Pythagoras (famous for maths), who lived in the 6th century BC in Athens, was said to believe that one's soul was reincarnated in an animal. Thus it was a sin to shed blood or eat meat. Also, like the Egyptian priests, he did not eat beans. An ancient lore was: boil a bean and expose it to moonlight for a proper number of nights, and you have – blood. The first recorded mention of bread was at the Siege of Tyre in 332 BC. Drops of blood trickling out from the besieging soldiers' bread were regarded as a good omen, and thereafter they succeeded in storming and destroying the city.

The occurrence of 'bleeding bread' (Figure 2) – especially that used as the 'host' for the communion service was obviously a major and recordable event. As the bread was often stored in damp medieval churches, it provided a good medium for bacterial growth. The appearance of drops of blood when a loaf was broken at a service must have seemed miraculous, and an event worthy of recording. Gaughran found 35 such reports – the first being in Alsen, Denmark in 1169 AD. 'The priest, stricken with fear' took the bleeding host to the bishop, who prophesied trouble ahead. Indeed 14 days later the country was invaded, and churches overthrown.

The most famous incident on record is of the 'Mass of Bolsena', which took place in 1263. The priest doubted the truth of the transubstantiation of the host into the body of Jesus, but as he

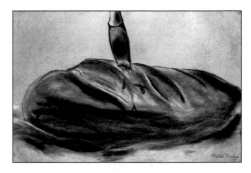

Figure 2   Bleeding bread (Martin Harding)

was blessing it drops of blood fell onto his robe. The Pope (Urban IV) issued a Papal Bull in 1264 to order 'Corpus Christi' as a feast day for the church. This is still observed, on the Sunday after Trinity Sunday. The event was used by Raphael in 1512–14 when he was decorating the 'Sala di Eliodoro' in the Vatican. His artistic license allowed his contemporary Pope (Julius II), to witness the miracle, together with his cardinals.

A more sinister aspect to the bleeding bread involved persecution of Jews, seen to be stabbing a host – in order to see the blood. Many (perhaps thousands) were said to have been slaughtered by the irate Christians.

Defining a germ

Padua in July 1819 was exceptionally warm and humid. In early July Dr Melo, curator of the botanic garden, was asked to 'purify' a house with a sick child, in which the 'polenta' (made from cornmeal) showed red spots – was this witchcraft? He reassured them it was not, and it did not recur. However the problem reappeared in a neighbouring farm where some left-over polenta, which had been kept in a drawer overnight, became covered in red spots. It was given to the hens, and a fresh batch prepared, which also developed the spots, as did some soup prepared for the children. Subsequent fasting and prayer did not protect a boiled hen kept in a locked kitchen cupboard from developing the spots. Rumours spread that a supernatural power had wreaked vengeance on the family because they hoarded corn in the previous year's famine. The entire neighbourhood came rushing to see and stood open-mouthed, and trembling. The medical officer of health, Dr Setto, was able to reproduce the spots on polenta in his own house, and also in that of the local priest, disproving that this could only happen in the abode of a sinner. The phenomenon spread, so that by 24 August 100 houses were affected, and by September when the moist Sirocco wind was replaced by the dry wind from the South and the outbreak ceased, over 300 families had been affected.

The disturbance became so great that the police were forced to notice it and ask the university to investigate. Bartomoleo Bizio (Figure 3) was a pharmacy student at the time (later professor in Venice), and although in the midst of superstition and panic, like Dr Setto he did careful, scientific experiments. His work could be regarded as the first reported use of solid culture media for bacteria, as he reproduced the red spots on a cornmeal mush, so antedating use of potato by Schroeter, and nutrient agar by Robert Koch 60 years later for growing bacteria. Within eight hours red spots appeared and after 24 hours the entire surface was discoloured. He noted the effect of temperature and humidity on development of the spots, and also the role of hands in their transmission. He thought it was a fungus without a stalk, and named it *Serratia* – in honour of the Italian physicist Serafino Serrati, who was thought to have invented the steamboat, and *marcescens* meaning decay – because the colour faded.

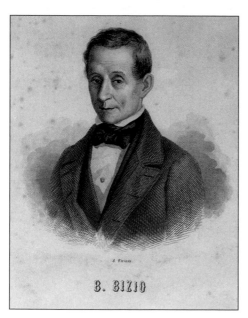

Figure 3   Bartomoleo Bizio (Andrea Bizio Gradenigo)

As time passed, Bizio was forgotten. In 1848, Dr Ehrenberg in Berlin touched the dry red spots

Table 1   Some names for *Serratia marcescens*

Serratia marcescens	Bizio	1823
Zoogalactia imetrofa	Sette	1824
Mucor sanguineus	DeCol	1824
Protococcus imetrophus	Menenghini	1838
Monas prodigiosa	Ehrenberg	1849
Bacteridium prodigiosum	Schroeter	1872
Bacilllus prodigiosus	Flugge	1886
Bacillus imetrophus	Trevisan	1887
Bacterium prodigiosum	Lehmann	1896
Erythrobacillus prodigiosus	Winslow	1920
Salmonella marcescens	Probram	1929
Chromobacterium prodigiosum	Topley and Wilson	1929

from some kitchen curtains onto the surface of a boiled potato, which in turn produced red spots that he transferred to white bread, and Swiss cheese. Microscopy showed small motile cells, which he thought were animal and called *Monas prodigiosum* (*Monas* – protozoon, and *prodigiosum* – miracle or omen). Once bacteriology took off with the availability of stains, microscopes, and culture media – the red colonies were a great attraction, and altogether 21 names are listed by Gaughran, ending in 1929, with *Chromobacterium prodigiosum* (Table 1). However by then Bizio's work had been rediscovered and *S. marcescens* was reinstated as the official name, although this took some time to be accepted.

Biological marker

The Houses of Parliament

Two years after 'the big stink', in which curtains soaked in chloride of lime had been hung to protect MPs from the smell of the Thames, the new Houses of Parliament opened (1860). These were spacious and fitted with a ventilation system. However, in 1903 members suffered an outbreak of influenza, and set up a committee to monitor the ventilation. Initial bacterial and chemical tests showed no excess of pollution, but 'this was not confirmed by the subjective tests of members own feelings'. So Dr MH Gordon was asked to investigate. He took two years, and his report (252 pages) makes fascinating reading (Gordon, 1906). Clearly my professor had read it.

Gordon concluded that the microbes in the debating chamber air were either brought in on the members' shoes (mainly faecal bacteria), or released from them during debates (streptococci). He used a culture of *C. prodigiosum* to help him decide which.

To test the shoes, sterile garden earth was mixed with a broth culture and some sterile sand to absorb excess moisture. A 1/4 lb tobacco tin with a perforated lid was used to sprinkle the gravel in New Palace Yard, 576 feet from the debating chamber. Culture plates were exposed for several hours at times when members moved around. The tests were repeated on five days, day 2 acting as an inadvertent negative control because 'the material was swept up within half an hour by a diligent sweeper'. There were other problems – members often jumped from their cabs directly on to pavement missing the gravel!! Anyway only two test plates grew the marker germ.

To test the breath, he read Shakespeare (Hamlet and Henry V) for one hour in a loud voice while standing at the dispatch box of an empty House of Commons, turning to address each corner of the house for 15 minutes with an audience of 200 Petri dishes. Two pairs of experiments were done – one with the ventilation off, and the other with it on. Each pair consisted of a control reading, followed by a test reading of the same material, before which he gargled with a culture of *C. prodigiosum*, and repeated after half an hour. The Petri dishes were exposed for one and a half hours. None were infected in the two control experiments, but in both tests around 25% of the plates grew the test organism (Figure 4). The number of colonies per plate was far greater in the test with the ventilation in use. This suggested that the ventilation was inadequate, and some modifications were put into place.

Flies and disease
Father had brought me up to beware of 'the filthy feet of the faecal feeding fly'. In 1910 Graham-Smith (lecturer in hygiene at Cambridge) reported a series of

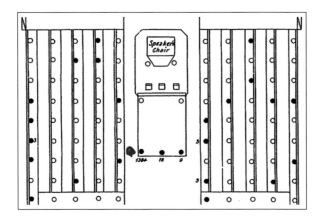

Figure 4   Results of cultures in the House of Commons (Gordon, 1906) red spot = dispatch box, black circles = positive culture plates (PSI License C2009000939)

ingenious experiments on the ability of house flies to spread bacteria, using *C. prodigiosum* as a marker (Graham-Smith, 1913). After a fly walked over a culture, the bacteria survived for up, to 48 hours on its legs and wings, but ingested bacteria survived in the gut for up to 17 days. Flies fed on contaminated syrup were placed in clean cages and then allowed to suck a crystal of brown sugar. The crystals were then dissolved in water and the

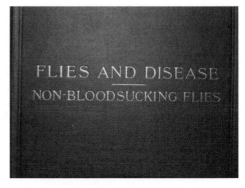

Figure 5   Flies and disease (Newsom)

solution cultured. Sugar lumps could be infected for up to two days (Figure 5).

Pathogenesis of infections
To show that hands could be important in spread of respiratory infection, US soldiers had their throats, lips and mouths sprayed with a culture of *C. prodigiosum*. This was then recovered from the hands, mess kits, and throats of non-infected soldiers. A more invasive set of tests was performed in 1940s Liverpool as part of an investigation of dental extractions and bacteraemia (McEntegart and Porterfield, 1949). Twenty-nine patients had *C. prodigiosum* painted on their gums before dental extractions, followed by a blood sample taken immediately afterwards. Twelve had positive blood cultures, so supporting the case for dental extractions as a cause of endocarditis.

Bioterrorism
In the days before germ warfare was outlawed, the US military used *S. marcescens* to see how they could deliver pathogens. The most unusual experiment was the release of the bacteria by US Navy ships into the ocean around San Francisco in 1950 and 1953. The waves produced aerosols, and bacteria were found in samples up to 80 meters inland. Yu noted: 'Public interest was ignited by the news that a San Francisco Hospital had experienced an outbreak of *S. marcescens* infections, including the first recorded case of endocarditis (fatal).'

Human infection
The first recorded human infection occurred in a patient with bronchiectasis reported in 1913. He was thought to have haemoptysis, but on sputum microscopy no red cells were seen. Culture revealed a heavy growth of *Serratia*. Another dramatic manifestation was the 'red diaper syndrome' reported in the

infant whose father was a professor of genetics in Madison, Wisconsin. Naturally he suspected a new inborn error of metabolism, but eventually the colour was shown to be prodigiosin. The strain of *S. marcescens* involved was shown to be the same as that used to study aerosols in a nearby research laboratory

The first documented outbreak (in San Francisco) began in October 1950 (Wheat et al. 1951). It involved 11 patients – all of whom had urinary tract manipulation of some kind. Two had a bacteraemia – in one it was transient, and the other developed a fatal endocarditis. The authors did not know of the naval experiments, and had no ideas as to the source of the outbreak. Actually although the naval experiment was the same year, subsequent analysis showed the strains used were different.

Since then, aided by its resistance to antibiotics and disinfectants *S. marcescens* has become a common nosocomial organism. A recent outbreak involved patients in an intensive care ward becoming infected from a contaminated water tap. The HIS 1981 survey revealed that 0.8% of nosocomial urinary tract infections were caused by *S. marcescens* and a good review was published by Hejazi and Falkiner in 1997.

Conclusion

I am happy to say I had no ill effects from gargling with *C. prodigiosum*, but I would not do so today. It has evolved from a medieval mystery germ, through being an excellent aerobiology test organism to the antibiotic-resistant *S. marcescens* of today. At least Bizio's name has stuck, and he did incriminate *hands* in the spread. Sadly he has never had the kudos he deserved.

Acknowledgements

I am very grateful to Martin Harding for Figure 2, to Andrea Bizio Gradenigo for the picture of his great-great-grandfather, and to Proquest Information for Figure 4.

Further reading

Gaughren GRL. (1969) From superstition to science; the history of a bacterium. *Transactions of the New York Academy of Sciences* **31**: 3–24.

Yu VL. (1979) *Serratia marcescens*. Historical perspective and clinical review. *N Engl J Med* **300**: 887–93.

Gordon MH. (1906) *Report on an investigation of the ventilation of the debating chamber of the House of Commons*. HMSO: London.

Graham-Smith GS. (1913) *Flies in relation to disease*. Cambridge University Press: Cambridge.

McEntegart MG. Porterfield JS. (1949) Bacteraemia following dental extractions. *Lancet* **ii**: 596–8.

Wheat RP. Zuckerman A. Rantz LA. (1951) Infection due to Chromobacteria. *Archives of Internal Medicine* **88**: 461–6.

Hejazi A. Falkiner FR. (1997) *Serratia marcescens*. *Journal of Medical Microbiology* **46**: 908–12.

Chapter 26

Sterilisers and the development of sterile services part 1

Introduction

Many of the events described in this article about sterilisation occurred during my own working life. We must start with the four elements ... of which fire was well known to the ancients for purification. There is too much to be told about sterilisation in one instalment. so the second part of the story will appear in Chapter 27.

Early sterilisation

Aristotle recommended that the Greek army should use boiled water for drinking, and the early use of steam under pressure related to food. Denis Papin described his engine for softening bones' in 1681 (see Figure 1), while in 1870 Albert Fryer of Manchester patented an autoclave for processing canned food (see Figure 2). It was not only heated by live steam from a separate boiler, but also after sterilisation it was cooled by introduction of water at the same pressure as the steam to prevent distortion of the cans.

Both Pasteur – boiling his growth medium, and Lister using Pasteur's methods with 'boiled liqueur glasses' knew the value of heat for killing microbes in the 1860s, but neither

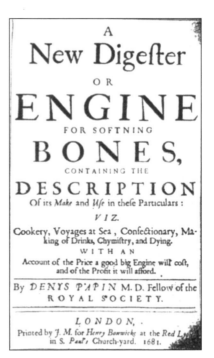

A

New Digeſter

OR

ENGINE

FOR SOFTNING

BONES,

CONTAINING THE

DESCRIPTION

Of its *Make* and *Uſe* in theſe Particulars :

VIZ.

Cookery, Voyages at Sea , Confectionary, Making of Drinks, Chymiſtry, and Dying.

WITH AN

Account of the Price a good big Engine will coſt, and of the Profit it will afford.

By *DENYS PAPIN* M. D. Fellow of the ROYAL SOCIETY.

LONDON, ·
Printed by *J. M.* for *Henry Bonwicke* at the *Red L* in S. *Paul's* Church-yard. 1681.

Figure 1 An 1861 advertisement for a 'bone digester' using steam

considered the problem of spores. In 1877 Pasteur said (to a surgical meeting): 'If I had the honour of being a surgeon, convinced as I am of the danger of germs scattered on surfaces, particularly in hospitals, not only would I use absolutely clean instruments, but after cleansing my hands with the greatest care, I would only use bandages and sponges which had previously been raised to a heat of 130–150°C'.

However it was Koch and his team who worked out the proper application of heat (both dry and moist) using sporeforming and non sporeforming bacteria, in addition to making many experiments on disinfectants (see Chapter 7).

Autoclaves

Little changed for 50 years after Koch. Autoclaves were by their nature very long-lasting pieces of equipment. Sterilising processes were in the 'cottage industry state' even in the 1950s. As a medical student I well remember the pleasures of coffee with the night nurse: a quiet chat while she filled a metal drum with cotton wool balls (removed from a roll) ready to be sent down for sterilising next day. The students also 'sterilised' their syringes in the ward boiler before the daily round of venepunctures.

The autoclave of that time was of a 'downward displacement' type (see Figure 3), which worked by letting steam in at the top of the chamber. As air

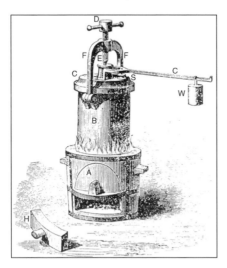

Figure 2   An early autoclave for processing canned food

is heavier than steam, it was pushed downwards and exhausted through a drain at the bottom of the chamber. Later models were fitted with a near to steam' valve in the exhaust, which would close when all the air had been removed, and allow the pressure in the vessel to build up. The removal of air was often aided by use of a simple 'venturi' pump, which consisted of steam passing through a nozzle across the exhaust line and so providing a partial vacuum. If a steam supply was not available, then the autoclave would be charged with water and used like a pressure cooker, heated by gas or electricity.

Dr Bowie in Edinburgh described the position in 1955 – About 90% of the sterilisers in use in Britain's hospitals and pharmacies were obsolete: they included representatives of all developmental stages in design since 1870. The Institute of Sterile Services Management's first President Sir James Howie, then Professor in Glasgow, took a major interest in the topic. He described how to examine and perform microbiological tests on autoclaves in the *Lancet* in 1956.

His account of testing five machines (all of which failed) commenced with instructions on how to handle the operating theatre sister tactfully before beginning! He felt that the metal drums were inadequate, and worried about re-contamination of the loads after sterilisation.

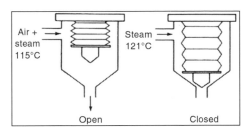

Figure 3   Early autoclave used a downward displacement method with a 'near to steam' valve in the exhaust that expanded to seal the autoclave once all the air was removed

The Nuffield Report

Enter the "yellow Peril". In 1958 the Nuffield Provincial Hospitals Trust published *Present Sterilising Practice in six hospitals* (See Figure 4). As a young trainee in pathology. I might not have been expected to take any interest in such a 'way out' review publication. However, one of the six was the London teaching hospital in which I was working!

This was a core document, because it fostered the concept of centralised reprocessing, which at that time only existed in plans for new hospitals and in military hospitals.

A team of three conducted what was in today's terminology an audit of sterile supply arrangements in one London teaching hospital, which happened to be ours, plus three provincial hospitals and two cottage hospitals. The team consisted of the scientist George Alder from Bristol, and two nurses. Miss AL Amsden and Miss DF Walker. They were directed by Brigadier Welch (later involved in the first Central Sterile Supply Department in the UK at Cambridge), and overseen by some eminent administrators. doctors and nurses of the time (Dr Revans. Dr Signy, Dr Darmady and Prof William Gillespie) who later became involved in founding the Central Sterilising Club.

Originally the audit was meant to be the introduction to a report on establishment of Central Sterile Supply Departments, but the team were so horrified by what they found that it was issued as a stand-alone document. The report has three main topics – wards, autoclaves and recommendations.

Studies of
Sterile Supply Arrangements
for Hospitals

PRESENT
STERILIZING PRACTICE
IN
SIX HOSPITALS

5s. net

THE NUFFIELD PROVINCIAL HOSPITALS TRUST
NUFFIELD LODGE, REGENT'S PARK, LONDON, N.W.1
1958

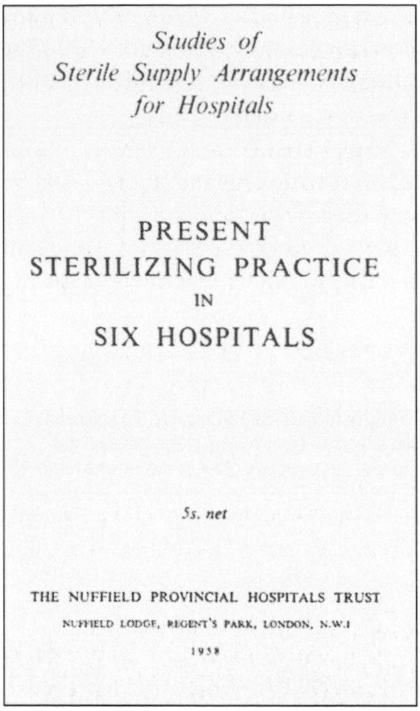

Figure 4 The influential Nuffield Report (Nuffield Trust)

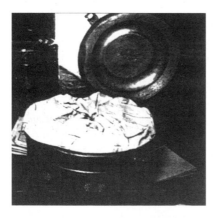

Figure 5 Over-packed metal drums full of dressings for autoclaving often prevented sterilisation (Nuffield report, Nuffield Trust)

Hot water sterilisers

Two main activities happened on the wards – as already noted, the nurses packed metal drums with swabs and dressings (see Figure 5). The 'duty (or clean utility) room contained a hot water steriliser (the ward boiler), storage for processed instruments (mainly in disinfectant), drums of sterile dressings, clean trolleys for laying up dressings, and a pair of cheatle forceps also in disinfectant for 'no touch' handling of the instruments. 'These clean utility rooms were not without drawbacks', wrote the team. 'Firstly many of them are nearer the ward than the sluice rooms so using them for disposal of dirty dressings was common.' The rooms were often cluttered and sometimes used as a general duty room so that telephoning went on. Opening the French windows allowed outside dust in to contaminate sterile material stored in front of them.

The hot water sterilisers were heated variously with gas, electricity or steam. On one occasion a nurse turned on the gas fully and set fire to the apron of the Sister who was standing alongside. None of the electrically operated sterilisers was fitted with a thermostat, timer, or rheostat. Thus they were difficult to operate correctly. I can well remember putting a bowl and syringe on top of another bowl that had been put in previously by a nurse. She removed her bowl almost immediately with the probability of it having been contaminated from the newer one. In fact even without the last in/first out situation, the team found that immersion rarely lasted for the recommended five minutes. In five of the hospitals hard water created problems. The photograph shown in Figure 6 shows a stainless steel measure after only five months of use. The team commented that stainless steel was used to provide a smooth surface; it could not be good practice to allow it to be so roughened.

The use of the metal containers for autoclaves created problems. The team found syringes in sealed metal boxes impervious to steam, and many defective drums. The drum was provided with a system whereby perforations – particularly in the top and bottom – were provided to allow the downward flow of steam and removal of air. The holes could be sealed after use by a slider that moved a sealing plate across them.

At the best of times, the steam penetration would be slow. If the drum was improperly packed, e.g. with too much material, or with a steam impenetrable liner, then steam could not penetrate – nor could it if someone forgot (as did happen from time to time) to open the holes or to place the drum in the autoclave so that the steam could pass through from top to bottom.

All in all, the team regarded the drum as an unsatisfactory piece of equipment, the replacement of which was long overdue. They noted that the Cambridge Military Hospital at Aldershot had used cardboard boxes among other things to meet the problems of the Suez crisis. The team did further research into cardboard boxes, which they noted allowed steam penetration better than a drum, and provided excellent protection to bacterial contamination of the contents after sterilisation.

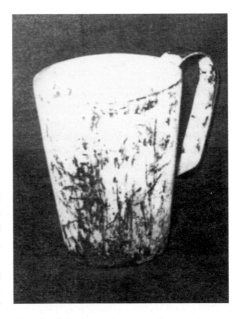

Figure 6   A stainless steel measure after several months of 're-sterilising' in a hot water 'steriliser' showing considerable crusting and damage (Nuffield report, Nuffield Trust)

Autoclave management

The other main topic of the audit was of the autoclave management. As will be seen, this struck home very much at our hospital. The autoclaves were run by a variety of staff. In one hospital a retired nursing sister appeared for two afternoons a week, and on other days nursing staff operated the autoclaves. In most other cases the attendants were male hospital porters responsible usually to the head porter, and sometimes to the theatre sister. In one hospital the porter was 'inclined to feel that he owed allegiance to the matron, but this was mainly because he also drove the nurses' bus'.

Thus it was not surprising that many of the failures of sterilising were attributed to the attendants rather than the equipment. In turn many people (myself included) did not fully understand how to operate autoclaves properly. Often the blame could be laid at the foot of the administration in failing to provide any education on the topic, or define a line management.

Most of the autoclaves were double-ended so that the packed drums could be fed in on one side and sterile drums removed and stored on the other. Sadly the report showed a photo of our steriliser attendant about to remove drums from the wrong side, standing beside a notice stating 'Sterile drums must not be taken out this side'. As a matter of interest, half the drums in the photograph are on their side, so air removal would be less efficient. The team reported that only eight of 17 autoclaves tested were working properly In our case there must have been a leaky door seal. As a result the air was never fully removed from the autoclave, so the near-to-steam valve remained open. In order to build up the pressure, a valve in the exhaust pipe was shut manually.

Premature closure of a chamber drain was in fact the commonest cause of autoclave failure noted by the team. An open drain was essential, 'otherwise the residual air cannot escape'.

Monitoring performance

Monitoring autoclave performance was a problem. All autoclaves had pressure gauges, and eight of those tested had pressure recorders, although one was out of action. In one machine the chart had been re-used so many times it was illegible. Measurement of temperature was a different matter.

Only five autoclaves had a thermometer in the chamber drain – in two of these taking a reading meant getting down on hands and knees, while a third had a broken thermometer. Thus only two autoclaves of the 17 tested had a proper thermometer. Occasional bacteriological tests were done. In our case in accordance (I now know) with Koch's practice, we used earth from the local graveyard as a test material.

The team concluded that most of the autoclaves tested were capable of sterilisation if they were properly set up and operated. They were strongly in favour of cardboard boxes rather than drums. However, their prime recommendation, which was a whole paragraph set out in capital letters, related to management structure. It was essential to replace the current *laissez faire* approach by a structure in which there was defined responsibility for hospital sterile services, proper equipment and proper training.

Outcomes of the report

While the situation did not change overnight, the hospitals concerned certainly changed some practices immediately. Our autoclaves were serviced, fitted with thermometers and were operated correctly from then on. It was, however, some years before a proper sterile supply service appeared.

The Nuffield Foundation did produce a second report on provision of sterile services, and they were also involved in prototype Central Sterile Supply Departments at Addenbrooke's Hospital in Cambridge and later at Musgrave Park in Belfast, and the Scottish service.

The year 1960 saw me joining the army, so I missed the setting up of The Central Sterilising Club out of which (eventually) grew the Institute of Sterile Services Management (now the Institute of Decontamination Sciences).

However, I have the programme for its second meeting, which was held in Cambridge in December 1960. Dr Gleeson White – my predecessor as Consultant microbiologist – gave me his copy complete with his opening lecture (see Figure 7). The Cambridge Central Sterile Supply Department had been open for six months.

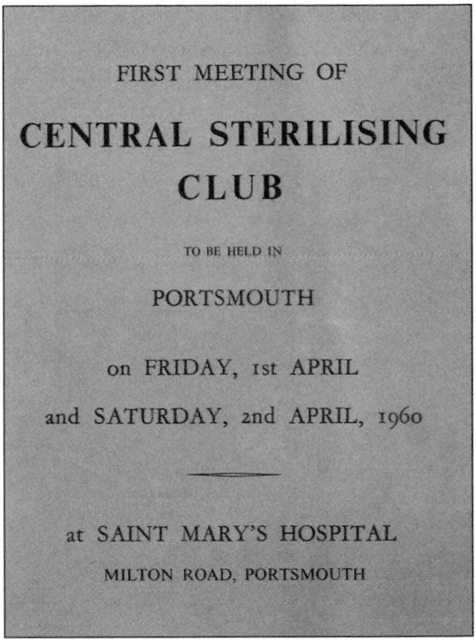

FIRST MEETING OF

CENTRAL STERILISING CLUB

TO BE HELD IN

PORTSMOUTH

on FRIDAY, 1st APRIL

and SATURDAY, 2nd APRIL, 1960

at SAINT MARY'S HOSPITAL

MILTON ROAD, PORTSMOUTH

Figure 7   The central sterilising club was the first UK 'infection control group'. It still provides a cross-disciplinary approach to the topic

The wards had been frightened about the loss of their sterilisers, and worried about the reliability of supplies. However by going gradually at it a ward at a time, and concentrating on good public relations, the service was settling down.

Developments

Outstanding questions (well advanced for 1960) included disposable equipment and disposal of disposables, use of ethylene oxide (a contentious topic for years), topical fluids, and responsibility for the equipment. In parallel with this, the Medical Research Council set up a working party to look at autoclaves. Their report stimulated the British Standards Institute to set standards for the forerunners of today's autoclaves. Dr Bowie and Mr Dick described their test: heat sensitive tape became available. The Department of Health set up various departments in the supplies and engineering divisions concerned with sterilisers (now coalesced into the Medicines and Healthcare products Regulatory Agency (MHRA)).

Things were looking well set. Then came the Devonport disaster, which in turn produced the 'Clothier report' and did much to stimulate Good Manufacturing Codes. All these things will be discussed in the next chapter.

Acknowledgement
I am very grateful to Dr Michael Scruton for help with the historical aspects of this article, and for the details of Papin's Digester. I am grateful to the Nuffield Provincial Hospitals Trust for Figures 4, 5 and 6.

Chapter 27
Sterilisers and the development of sterile services part 2

Introduction

Chapter 26 ended more or less in 1960, with the Medical Research Council (MRQ/British Standards Institute (BSI) advisers looking into improvement in autoclaves and me departing for Hong Kong to work in the Army Hospital. Like the last article – perhaps even more so – this will be a personal account of events, rather than an unbiased or comprehensive story. The army laboratory had its own sterilisers (gas-fired, milk-churn type): and I inherited a going concern, both technician and standard operating practices, so for a while all went well. Then two upsets occurred, which although I did not know it, were symptomatic of widespread problems, namely the need to re-use needles, and sterilisation of fluids.

Re-use of needles

The army suddenly ordered yellow fever vaccination for all soldiers. There were 10,000 of them in Hong Kong, and only one qualified vaccinator – me. When I needed a day out I set off into the country to a suitable army camp bearing my vaccine, and my supply of around five needles, together with an oil bath and five syringes. After each injection the needle (syringe attached) was plunged into the oil bath (140°C) for the required time, then re-used.

However, re-use of needles had indeed already created outbreaks of jaundice in places such as diabetic clinics. I later found out that the MRC had issued their Memorandum *The Sterilisation, Use and Care of Syringes* in 1945 (see Figure 1) then revised it in 1962. The Nuffield Trust had preceded the 'yellow peril' with the report *Planning and Organisation of Central Syringe Services* (1957).

The MRC recommended dry heat sterilisation with syringes and needles assembled in aluminium tubes (as steam could not penetrate into the syringe), and to my horror specifically warned against using hot oil. The oil bath was an army approved method at the time I used it. All I can say is that no one turned up to our hospital with jaundice after being vaccinated, but

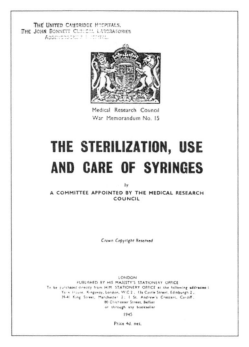

THE UNITED CAMBRIDGE HOSPITALS.
THE JOHN BONNETT CLINICAL LABORATORIES
ADDENBROOKE'S HOSPITAL

Medical Research Council
War Memorandum No. 15

THE STERILIZATION, USE AND CARE OF SYRINGES

by

A COMMITTEE APPOINTED BY THE MEDICAL RESEARCH
COUNCIL

Crown Copyright Reserved

LONDON
PUBLISHED BY HIS MAJESTY'S STATIONERY OFFICE
To be purchased directly from H.M. STATIONERY OFFICE at the following addresses:
York House, Kingsway, London, W.C.2; 13a Castle Street, Edinburgh 2;
39-41 King Street, Manchester 2; 1 St. Andrew's Crescent, Cardiff;
80 Chichester Street, Belfast
or through any bookseller

1945

Price 4d. net.

Figure 1   The Medical Research Council published this memorandum in 1945, following outbreaks of syringe-spread jaundice (PSI License C2009000939)

now I realise how lucky I was (or the soldiers were). Today these problems are old history thanks to widespread use of disposables, although of course needle disposal brings other problems with it.

Sterilisation of fluids

The other problem arose when the army issued an edict saying 'no more local production of intravenous fluids'. I was very relieved that Private Fox (doing National Service) no longer had to make up the hospital IV fluids.

However, the replacements (from Army Stores, UK) were one litre bags sealed into giving sets and needles as a single unit. If you wished to give more than one litre, you had to put up a new drip (I later found out that these bags had been stockpiled for the event of nuclear war, when if you needed more than one litre, you were probably unsalvageable).

The clinical doctors said to me: 'We are not using these – please continue making the fluids in bottles as before.' So I did, but with one difference – I no longer had a supply of new suba-seals'. These red rubber bungs had a circle on the top, divided into four sectors (labelled 1, 2, 3 and 4). In my ignorance I assumed that a needle could be put through each in turn – four times usage. Fortunately for me the Army had another practice – to examine each bottle of IV fluid in a special light box before using it.

Three months later I was handed a bottle of saline containing a large fungus ball. A rapid tour of ward stores revealed four more unused bottles in the same condition, and I closed production forthwith. I later learnt that fungal spores can quite often penetrate where bacteria cannot, and cracks in the glass of bottles (usually around the rim) may even be enough to allow penetration of fungal spores.

Provision of IV fluids in the NHS was a pharmacy job (one of the original Central Sterile Supply Department (CSSD) Managers was a pharmacist). In some hospitals this was done 'on site' and in others commercial products were used. The CSSD remained involved in production of sterile water for operating theatres. Fluids autoclaves were of the large downward displacement type. However, the cycle time needed to be longer because steam only condenses on the surface of a container, and the heat is then transferred gradually throughout the liquid in it by a thermo-syphon.

This was brought home to me by two incidents. Firstly, back in London after my army days were over, I had asked for a five litre container of culture medium to be sterilised. The container was put into the laboratory autoclave and when the cycle was finished it was left to cool overnight. Next morning the liquid was cloudy and contained a good growth of bacteria. Thus it had never reached sterilising temperature, but had achieved a nice temperature for growth of the bacteria from the original powder. Secondly, when I tested a decontamination cycle on a new laboratory autoclave in Cambridge by putting a thermocouple into a bottle of medium, I found that it only reached sterilising temperature by the time the autoclave cycle finished.

So I knew that sterilising liquids in an autoclave could provide problems. However, like most people I never thought to question commercially prepared IV fluids. After all the label on the bottle stated 'sterile'.

The Devonport incident

Then came the Devonport disaster. The paper written by Dr Meers and colleagues in the Lancet (see Figure 2) had a more sedate title.

On 1 to 3 March 1972 the two surgeons in Devonport noted a series of untoward reactions in their patients, which worried them enough to stop all surgery and to cease using any intravenous fluids containing glucose (because all patients affected had received such fluids). Five patients died. All had collapsed after receiving 5% dextrose. Of the 17 unused bottles recovered 14 grew bacteria (not all of the same type), in counts of up to one million/ml. Many bottles were seen to be cloudy. The bottles all appeared to come from the same sub-batch, manufactured by Evans Medical. Although the labels indicated the

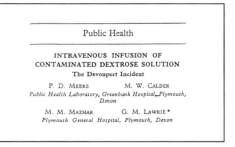

Figure 2   Dr Meers and colleagues published their review of the Devonport incident, which claimed the lives of five patients in 1972

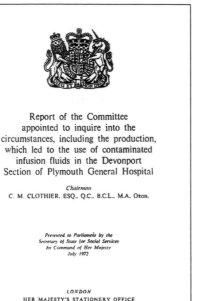

Report of the Committee
appointed to inquire into the
circumstances, including the production,
which led to the use of contaminated
infusion fluids in the Devonport
Section of Plymouth General Hospital

Chairman
C. M. CLOTHIER, ESQ., Q.C., B.C.L., M.A. Oxon.

Presented to Parliament by the
Secretary of State for Social Services
by Command of Her Majesty
July 1972

LONDON
HER MAJESTY'S STATIONERY OFFICE
24p net
Cmnd. 5035

Figure 3   The official 'Clothier' report of the Devonport incident revealed gross inadequacies in sterilisation processes (PSI License C2009000939)

sub-batch number (and so the actual autoclave used), this was not recorded by the staff in patients notes, so final proof was circumstantial.

The report of the Government Committee of Inquiry into the incident – the 'Clothier' report (see Figure 3), makes chilling reading. Of the relevant sub-batch placed in autoclave number four, about one-third of the bottles failed to reach sterilising temperature, due to retention of air. There was evidence of this failure because the recording thermometer failed to indicate a rise in temperature. This was however ignored (in contravention of the operating procedures) on the grounds that the recording thermometers had a history of unreliable operation. The chargehand gave evidence that other autoclaves had given low temperature readings in the past, and the procedure then was to check the steam trap and summon the engineer. If the steam trap was working satisfactorily, the temperature recorders were regarded as faulty. This was obviously a dangerous situation. The media followed it closely and a newspaper reported one of the staff as saying: 'I know when she (the steam trap) gives trouble, because she whistles, then I gives her a good kick!' The autoclaves must have been working very badly because the types of bacteria found by Dr Meers in the fluids were of the normal heat-sensitive type.

Although this incident did not involve CSSDs, and was concerned with production of sterile fluids, it was highly relevant. The Committee made detailed recommendations to the Medicines Commission, stressing in particular the need for clear labelling and recording of batch numbers, and the use of plastic containers instead of bottles. All in all, the incident served as a basis for the subsequent production of codes of good manufacturing practice. It also stimulated the idea of using thermocouples inside dummy bottles to monitor the load, and the production of master records for different types of fluid loads.

Dressings sterilisers

The 'yellow peril' had highlighted the dangers of using downward displacement autoclaves for dressings. The MRC working party on pressure steam sterilisers published three reports in the *Lancet* between 1959 and 1964, then disbanded – its work done, although many of the members had transferred their expertise to the BSI, and standards for high vacuum dressings sterilisers had emerged.

The first report echoed many of the findings of the yellow peril, pointing out the dangers of using downward displacement sterilisers for dressings, in that air removal even in properly maintained machines was problematic. High vacuum machines were much to be preferred. They also discussed steam quality, and criticised the practice of maintaining the jacket at a higher temperature than the chamber as likely to contribute to superheat (when my predecessor in East Anglia visited a mental hospital, he was puzzled by the rusty appearance of the steam, and asked why the autoclave loads did not come out stained. 'They used to', came the reply, 'but now we only put the steam in the jacket!').

Common faults addressed were damage to materials (some cycles were up to five hours long), wet loads, steam quality and non-condensable gases, autoclave and drum loading, re–contamination of the load after processing, and the use of untrained staff.

Installation and maintenance came under scrutiny. Topics highlighted included siting, steam quality, drains, inefficient venting (waste steam may be discharged into the room, not only causing damage to walls and ceilings, but also the noise may disturb the surgeon), and inefficient design so that the back of the chamber may not be usable (for a long cylinder). Poor maintenance of temperature and pressure recorders, leaky gaskets, poor door hinges (potentially lethal) and blocked discharge channels were all noted.

Besides encouraging use of high vacuum machines, the report concluded that the underlying factor contributing to inefficient sterilisation was ignorance, which the group (all doctors) attributed to the lack of any single member of the medical staff having final responsibility for selection and use of equipment, and of training operators properly.

The MRC second report in 1960 continued to encourage use of high vacuum machines (see Figure 4), and to emphasise the greater throughput. One of the members, Professor Wells, reported on the introduction of a high vacuum machine into a 650-bed hospital. Previously the weekly load had been 1000 dressing drums and 140 glove drums. A 72ft^3 autoclave was used with cycles lasting 160 minutes for drums, and 90 for gloves. Two full-time operators were needed, covering between them 0700 to 2100 hours per day (less at weekends). The replacement autoclave required slightly longer (0700 to 2220), but still only needed two operators, and was only 3.5ft^3 in capacity. The *Lancet* commented that smaller, more efficient machines would easily repay their cost, especially if hospitals got together to rationalise their sterilising procedures into central sterilising departments.

By the time the MRC published their final report in 1964, the high vacuum machines were making an impact. Three topics had emerged. Firstly was the 'small load effect', the concentration of residual air in a small load in a machine not functioning properly. Next was perhaps the first readily available publication of the Bowie-Dick test, and thirdly the comment that high vacuum sterilisers had proved satisfactory for sterilisation of unwrapped instruments and bowls. The working party concluded that its work was finished and referred readers to the relevant British Standards and to HTM 10, which had been published by the Ministry of Health in 1960.

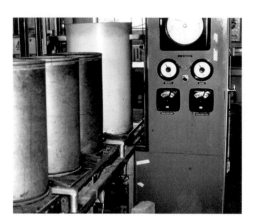

Figure 4   An automated high-vacuum steriliser of the 1960s, made to standards set in the Medical Research Council report of 1960 (Newsom)

When I entered onto the UK scene in 1967, I found myself as the adviser on sterilisation matters in East Anglia. This involved advice on the planning of a rational CSSD provision, on setting up CSSDs, purchase of autoclaves and for autoclave testing. I still have my single Servoscribe recorder and copper/constantam wire. This was quite a daunting job for a microbiologist. Then in the 1970s I became a member of the British Standard (BS) Committee chaired by Dr Bowie, charged with the job of revising the standards. Graham Ayliffe was also a member. It was a long and tedious job – just as we had come to a conclusion about something, the technology changed and we had to start again. Eventually I gave up, as I had become Chairman of a separate BS Committee. The BS did eventually produce revisions, but was soon involved in European Standards – which was a whole new ball game.

One plus point of attending the BS were the people. From Sheffield came Sid Gibbons, one of the first NHS steriliser engineers. Bearing in mind the variable quality of hospital staff, the Regional Engineer seemed like an excellent idea to me. I tried hard for one in East Anglia, but all I achieved was four sets of highly expensive ten-point recorders – one for each major hospital in the region. However, suddenly the Department of Health decided that Regional Engineers were in and all was well. My role changed to occasional teaching on the Falfield courses, and to keeping an eye on our own CSSDs.

Later years

In the 1970s life became more settled. CSSDs were present and correct, and reasonable high-vacuum machines were installed – like the automatic Sanderson we used at Bury St Edmunds (see Figure 4). Proper packaging materials became available, and it was realised that stainless steel could be replaced by polypropylene. Derek Booth at Warwick SASCO had a major role in the development of plastic holloware. This was a major improvement on stainless steel, although sometimes not without problems. Sid Gibbons did a lot to teach people about steam quality and the dangers of superheat, both due to the steam and the presence of a large dry load in the autoclave. As the deforming point of the polypropylene is only 139°C, a few degrees of superheat may create problems (Figure 5).

Disposable equipment

Later of course came the introduction and widespread use of disposable plastic items. One such – a pair of forceps with a patent hinge – was introduced by ICI costed as a disposable (see Figure 6). It was made of polypropylene and would actually withstand 100 sterilisation cycles. The ICI technical officer came to tell me that they could make them turn black, or explode in the autoclave, to ensure disposal. Actually, although a very robust piece of equipment, this is now consigned to the history books.

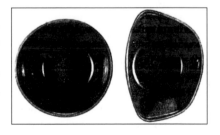

Figure 5 'Dished' polypropylene bowls before and after autoclaving showing 'superheat' (Newsom)

My involvement with sterilisers in later years became less and less. Computer controls came in, together with much more sophisticated monitoring systems. I did note with amusement one day when our local engineer pressed the wrong button on his handheld programmer, and the result was that the laboratory autoclave

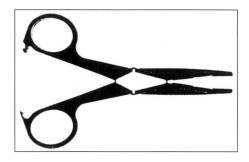

Figure 6   Polypropylene forceps introduced by ICI were meant (and priced) to be disposable, but could withstand 100 sterilisation cycles (Newsom)

'crashed' in the middle of a cycle. It needed the maker's engineers to get the door open. All of which makes me wonder what this millennium holds in store.

Postscript

Chapter 27 was originally written in 1999. Little did I know what was to follow. A quick scan of the Brussels Gare du Midi bookstore in May 2001 to find suitable reading for Eurostar revealed a paperback: *La Scandale du Cidex* illustrated by a photo of a surgical team. A compulsive purchase. However the content was not about hazards to healthcare workers, but the doomsday scenario of what happens when unsterile instruments are used for invasive procedures. The millennium bug caused the scandal.

To avoid problems in the factory (in the UK) the glutaraldehyde dilution plant was closed down over the New Year 2000 and the tank normally used for concentrated glutaraldehyde was filled with water to prevent corrosion. The new year's day operator didn't know. Thus some or all of the first batch (3.300 × 51 containers) of the new millennium (Batch 0001), which was mainly sold in Belgium, was made by adding water (2.2%) to water. It arrived in Belgium in February and was used for sterilising surgical/endoscope equipment. On 13 March a hospital reported a failed activity check (bandelette).

This was assumed to be an indicator failure, but a fortnight later a second Belgian hospital reported inactivity of the same batch of Cidex, and by early April the manufacturers were warning Belgian pharmacies to withdraw what was left of the batch. The book explores the consequences of this situation, which resulted in 34,870 people having procedures with presumptively unsterile instruments.

A later Belgian Government report provided follow up on 24,832 patients – 18,315 of whom had a blood test for HBV, and 19,256 for HCV. The incidence of positives was no different to the general population. Eight patients had a bacteraemia, but none developed tuberculosis. Thus surprisingly results bear out the conclusions of others that transmission of HBV or HCV by endoscopy is low.

Nonetheless a salutary story – one can have very advanced technology – but it all depends on humans. A fitting end to my book.

Further reading

Debacker N. Carsauw H. *Suivi Epidemiologiqae de L' incident Cidex Lot No 0001*. Brussels; Institut Scientifique de la sante publique, IPH/EPI Reports No. 2001–010 (for those who can read French!).

Morris J. Duckworth GJ. Ridgway GL. Gastro-intestinal endoscopy decontamination failure and the risk of blood borne viruses: a review. *J Hosp Infect* 2006; **63**: 1–13.

Index